Hormonal Harmony

Publisher: Susanne Christina Haegele, Paris, France.
Copyright: ©Susanne Christina Haegele, Paris, France, 2020.

This text is an adapted translation of the French original *Hormones en Harmonie*, Paris 2019.
Adapted and translated by Susanne Haegele with Sarah Burgess.

Printed by Ingram. Print on demand.
ISBN 978-2-9574040-0-1 for the Print Edition
ISBN 978-2-9574040-1-8 for the e-Book.

Price in GBP: 18 GBP.
Legal deposit: under way.

Note to the reader: the postures and practical tips presented in this book are meant for persons in good health. If you suffer from any specific ailment or predisposition, check with a yoga teacher and your general practitioner before practicing them. The publisher declines any responsibility for any injuries derived from the postures and practical tips offered in this book. Furthermore, the information about essential oils does not in any instance replace the advice and prescriptions of a medical professional.

Photo credits:
Heather Whitehouse pp. 8, 12, 14, 19, 24.
Adèle Chrétien (Yellothere) pp. 50, 96, 101.
Cecilia Cristolovean (@yogaandphoto) for all the yoga sequences.
Adobe stock on pp. 11, 16-17, 20, 22-23, 80.
Portraits of the 6 co-authors: their private property.
Anatomical illustrations: Elena Jarmosh.

The yoga clothes worn in this book are from *Shambhala*, Spain. The outfits worn in the Youtube videos are from *Devi Active YogaWear by Mirjam*, Brazil. Both brands are eco-conscious and socially engaged.

Hormonal Harmony

A NATURAL GUIDE TO WOMEN'S WELLBEING

Susanne Haegele

Table of contents

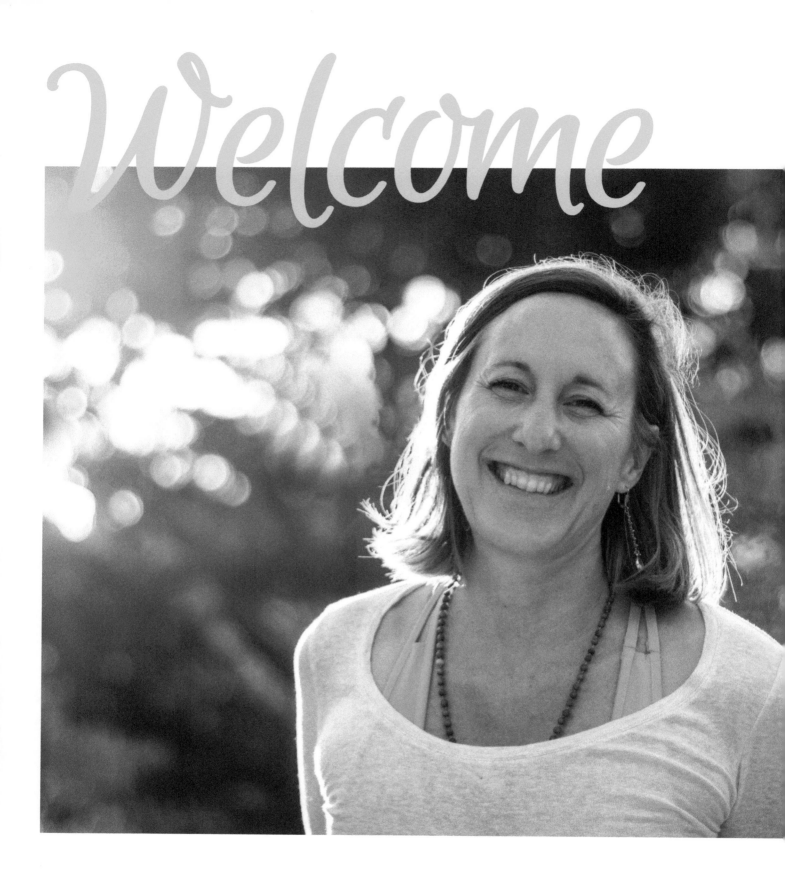

Welcome

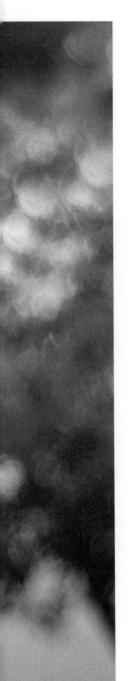

Ours is a fascinating time to be a woman. In the West, Women's Lib', sexual education, the contraceptive pill, and hormone treatments for fertility or menopause, give the impression that modern women are comfortable in their own skin, well informed, and thriving. Many taboos around the female body are openly mentioned at last. The film *Period. End of Sentence*, about issues around menstruation in an Indian village, even won an Oscar in 2019, and on social platforms women are using the hashtag *#metoo* to name and shame macho behaviour that has become unacceptable at last.

And yet, what a Pandora's box opened when I began to specialise in yoga for women's health! Exhaustion, anxiety, premenstrual syndrome, hypothyroidism, endometriosis, fertility issues, cancer, vaginal dryness, and urinary incontinence are just a sample of the worries women share with me every day, be it during the workshops I teach, or when I meet up with friends, former work colleagues, and family members. As soon as I mention the subject, women of all ages confide in me with their personal stories.

It is always my pleasure to share with them what I have learnt during my yoga training, by reading numerous specialists' books, and thanks to my encounters with other professionals focusing on natural approaches to health, such as the ones who kindly joined me in creating the book you are now reading.

One thing is as certain as it is surprising: practically every woman I know – some of whom lead a very healthy life – regularly suffer from some kind of trouble at the physical or mental / psychological level.

Luckily, there are many simple, natural and affordable solutions available to help women restore their balance. I present some of them in this book, which by no means aims to list them all, but summarises the questions which seem to preoccupy many of us, and offers tried and tested answers.

This book certainly does not claim to be able to heal a serious illness, and does not replace a medical diagnosis and treatment.

Yet we give you important keys for your physical and emotional wellbeing, because today's women want to understand what is happening to them, make informed decisions, and take ownership of their wellbeing.

Every day gives you the opportunity to look after yourself, be it whilst you are undergoing medical treatment, or, ideally, preventatively. Welcome to our circle, and welcome to your body.

How to use this guide?

I chose to organise this book around themes, rather than following a chronological path from the first menstruation to life after menopause, because some questions reappear at different times in a woman's life. Also, you can lay the foundations for feeling well in later life many years in advance, as long as you know how to do it!

What do a perimenopausal woman, an adolescent experiencing puberty, a pregnant woman, and a young mother all have in common? Hormonal fluctuations. Even though their circumstances differ significantly, some symptoms seem strangely similar: skin rashes, mood swings, digestive issues, thrush, fatigue, unstable joints, unpredictable libido…

To find out what is going on, we will travel "downwards" through the body. Our exploration of the feminine body will take us from the head to the pelvic floor. Depending on your current situation, you can choose to go directly to the index, to find the pages where a specific question is discussed, or go with the flow of the book to allow yourself to be surprised.
I would also encourage you to check out the commented bibliography, to find other books which go into more detail regarding the particular issue you are interested in.

The yoga poses I chose are relatively simple and brief ones, which can safely be practised at home.
On www.susanne-haegele.com and the Youtube channel of the same name, you will find mini-videos showing how to get into and out of the postures, and how to do the massages.

You can find recordings of the meditations in English on my Youtube channel. If you understand French, you can also log into the French specialised yoga website www.myYogaconnect.fr for full classes of the four sequences with my explanations (the first two weeks of subscription are free).

When is the best time to practise yoga? For the active postures, it is better to wait at least two hours after a meal, meaning in the morning before breakfast, just before lunch, or in the evening before dinner. You could also do them just before bed if you can dine early (albeit the digestive sequence is bit too active for the evenings). Yoga postures and a full belly don't go well together, apart from the resting poses. NB: the postures marked with this symbol: X! are not appropriate for pregnant women.

A yoga mat is the only thing you need, and even that is optional for most postures. There is no need to wear a special outfit - the only reason I wear a tight jumpsuit in the photos and videos is so that you can clearly see the positioning of my body in each pose. What you do need is a calm, clean, well-aired space that is reasonably warm. Blankets and pillows will be useful for the restorative poses. If silence is uncomfortable for you, soft and relaxing background music will create the right atmosphere.

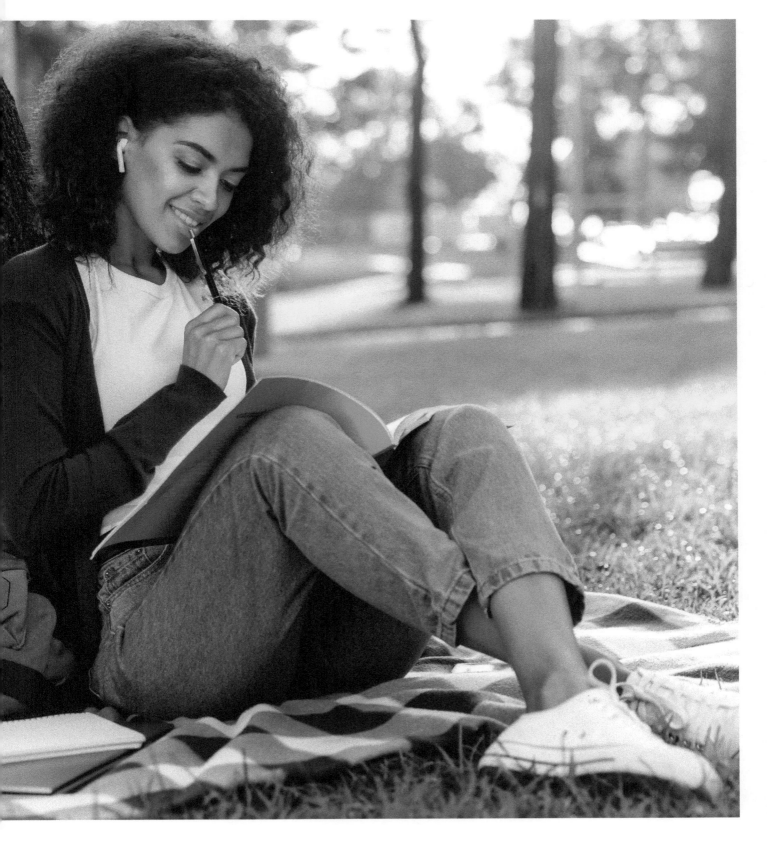

The 5 elements of women's wellbeing

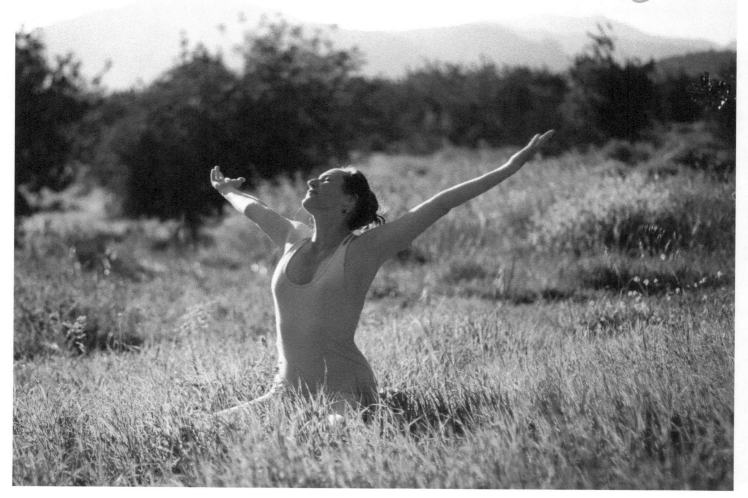

The human body has an impressive ability to regenerate and heal. A scratch that soon vanishes, or a torn nail that grows back, prove this daily on a small scale. **This constant striving for balance is called *homeostasis.*** So, how come we are not all perfectly healthy, physically and mentally, at least those of us who live under "normal" conditions, with a roof over our head and daily meals?

Do you realise that your body and mind are still, from an evolutionary point of view, those of a woman living in a hunter-gatherer tribe? Our lifestyle change is fairly recent: until approximately 12,000 years ago, before the transition to agriculture, humans made a living hunting and gathering. From an evolutionary perspective, this was yesterday. As far as our current Western lifestyle is concerned, created by industrialisation, then transformed again by the digital revolution, it only started a moment ago on the scale of humanity.

So, what has this got to do with my daily life and my health, you may ask?

Western scientists such as Jean Liedloff or Françoise Freedman, who have lived with tribal people in the South American jungle, have brought back fascinating accounts of a lifestyle which resembles that of our ancestors. Without ignoring the real dangers of life in the jungle, they describe calm, graceful, self-assured women, who go about their daily tasks serenely and in harmony with the world around them.

They are rarely alone, but neither are they confronted every day with a crowd of strangers in a confined setting. They receive help from their neighbours and family in case of an accident or when they give birth. Their children are raised by the entire village and learn by imitating adults. The various phases of a woman's life are no mystery to them, since they have had the chance to observe other female members of their tribe since childhood, and their way of life is similar to that of their ancestors. Elders are integrated into the community and respected for their wisdom. Since they carry loads on their heads, these women have a strong pelvic floor and strong back muscles, as well as good bones. Living outside, they breathe fresh air and do not lack vitamin D. Since they walk regularly, and sit cross-legged or squat, their legs are athletic and blood circulates well in their pelvic region, helping with good digestion and trouble-free menstruation.

Most of us have no plans to move to the jungle, and cannot even change jobs or way of life very easily, at least not straight away. The idea is therefore to bring back into our daily life the traditional moves, sensations, and rhythms of former times, so that our body can keep regenerating itself when confronted with life's small and large challenges.

Of course, this applies to men as much as it does to women, but women's situation is different from men's due to their hormonal cycle, the impact of potential motherhood and also the fact that they are amongst the very few mammals that experience menopause.

The most important thing to realise is therefore that we are cyclical, because of the hormonal fluctuations which return approximately every month, following a precise blueprint, from the first to the last menstruation, and even beyond. You may know this, but do you also know how to respect these cycles, and do you understand how important they are for your health?

Hormones are messages sent through the bloodstream towards the cells by certain glands, as a reaction to what our body perceives about the environment in which it finds itself.

Their mission is to help the body adapt as well as possible to any changes within this environment. It is as simple and as impressive as that, and it brings us back once more to our stone-age ancestor: to ensure her survival, she was only fertile in an adequate environment, and her metabolism slowed down to store fat reserves if the circumstances were perceived as hostile.

Any form of stress or perceived lack will cause a change in the hormonal messages. What is called a "dysfunction" is therefore actually often an adaptation. To ignore this reality means to deprive yourself of important keys to feeling well.

In practice, the following five elements are crucial for feminine wellbeing, at any age.

When a woman feels out of balance and seems to be "withering", there is often an imbalance in one (or several) of these areas:

- Movement
- Rest
- Digestion
- Disconnection
- Connection

Do some elements seem to contradict each other? Wait and see how they actually work together.

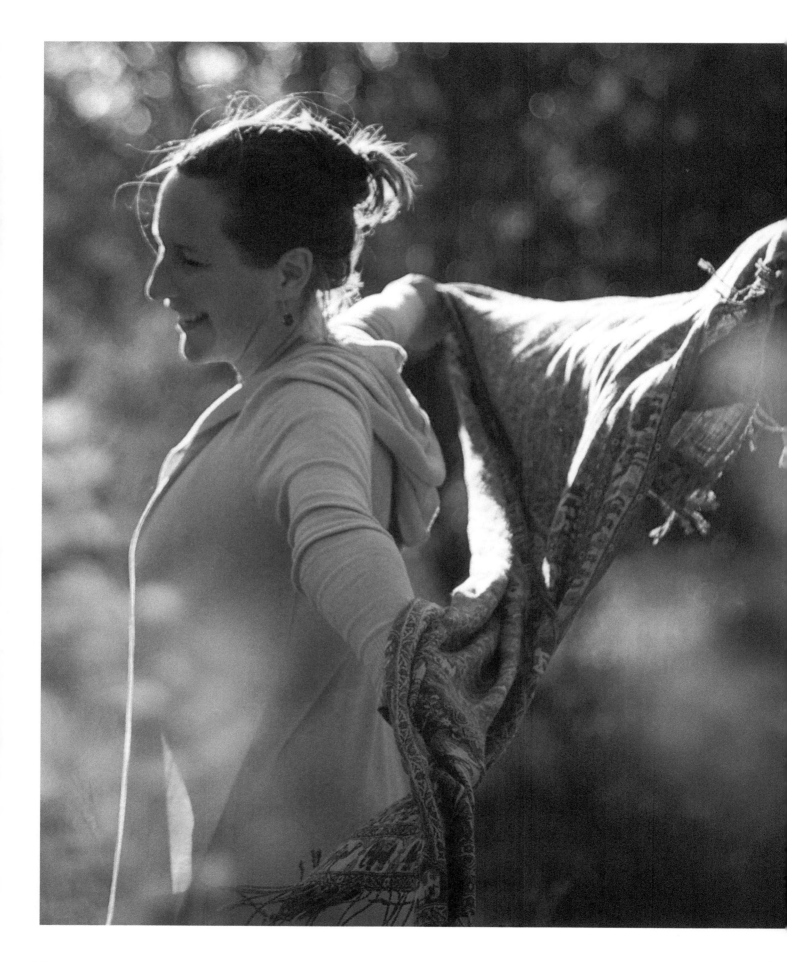

Movement

To make our lives easier and "save time", we have reduced our walking time and our manual labour, so that we now live mostly seated on chairs or sofas. As a consequence, the Western sedentary (meaning "seated" or "inactive") lifestyle has become a public health issue.

Some of us move too little, which, apart from excess weight gain, fragile bones, weak muscles and lack of oxygen, also deprives us of the mental relaxation induced by physical exercise. In addition women often suffer with "stagnation" (lack of blood and lymph circulation) in the legs and pelvis, which causes all kinds of trouble (painful periods, constipation, heavy legs…).
The lack of time or money to "get started" is often said to be the issue, but you can move at home, in your pyjamas!
I hope that the yoga sequences presented in this book are simple and short enough to make you want to try them at home. If you add a regular walk outside, or a short break to dance to your favourite music, this will be a big step in the right direction, and may already make a real difference.

On the other hand, some women tend to push themselves too hard, or move in a jerky or linear way, whereas women's bodies are built for a smooth and swinging step. Most of all, they cannot always summon the exact same amount of energy, depending on the phase of their menstrual cycle. If running marathons or playing tennis until you are panting makes you happy, it can be interesting for your wellbeing to add a few different moves to your sports practise. First and foremost, you will benefit from adding sufficient time to rest and recharge.

I have chosen moves and postures which can help to stretch or strengthen certain muscles which are important for your hormonal balance, such as the adductor muscles, the psoas and the pelvic floor. The moves also stimulate and massage certain organs, whilst helping to release tension.

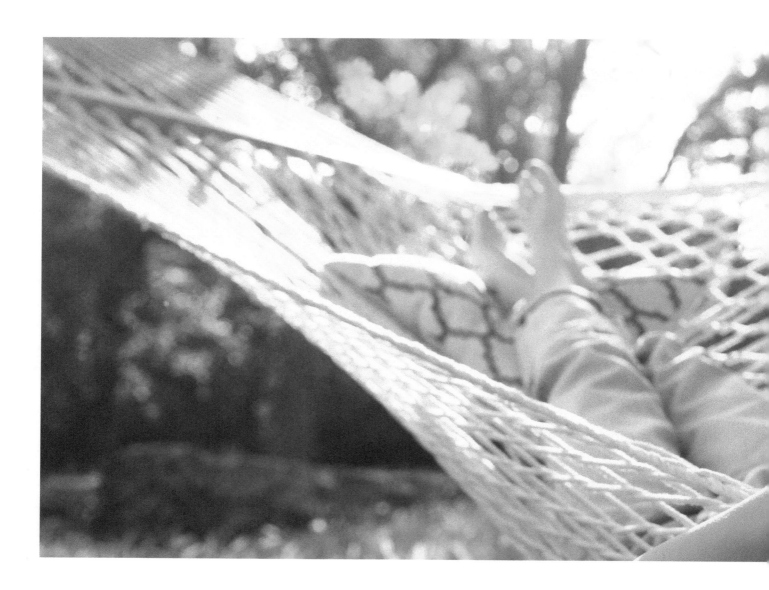

Rest

Almost all (Western) women have one thing in common: they need more quality rest, especially during their period, around the birth of their children, when life presents them with a big challenge, and during perimenopause. This means that the menstrual cycle, as well as different needs at various times in your life, should be taken into account.

In his bestseller *Sapiens*, historian Yuval N. Harari mentions the theory about the "abundant society" of nomadic hunter-gatherers. Apparently, their working life was much less intense than our modern one, with a greater variety of tasks and more time to chat and to celebrate.
Seen in this light, the chronic fatigue so many women suffer from is easier to understand!
Yet if you are able to settle in a pleasant position

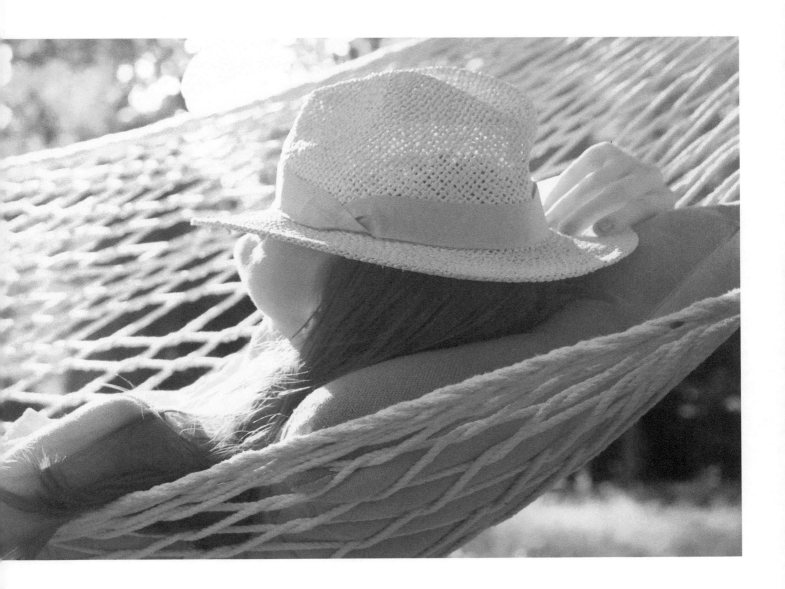

which does not compress your chest or your lower back, in silence, or with soft background music, focusing on nothing but your own breath, ten short minutes of quality rest will already regenerate you. Conversely, slouching on the sofa whilst watching a box set (as fascinating as the storyline may be!) cannot fulfil the same function: your nervous system is very excited by the plot (it cannot distinguish between a real event and an invented story) whilst your neck muscles and your spine suffer in the slouching posture.

Insomnia currently affects up to one third of the UK's population (defined as lack of sleep or poor quality sleep).[ii] Considering that the body regenerates at night, and our brain "cleans itself" only when we sleep, the consequences of insomnia are serious and long-lasting.

A good night's sleep is prepared beforehand by simple choices such as reducing stimulating substances, switching off all screens an hour before bed, or knowing how to **activate our parasympathetic nervous system**, which helps us to rest and regenerate.

To sleep well at night is essential, but does not replace taking short breaks, for example after a meal or upon returning from work.

Most people's natural biorhythm isn't synced with the average working day (plus a commute), and we often compensate for "energy slumps" by making choices which deplete the body over the long term.

The methods described in this book will help you activate those parts of your nervous system which help you relax and recharge.

Digestion

A good digestion is crucial, not just for our physical balance, but also for our emotional wellbeing. German medical student Giulia Enders, who wrote the bestseller *Gut: the inside story of our body's most under-rated organ*, brought to the attention of the general public what nutritionists and naturopathic practitioners have been telling us for a long time: excess weight, acne, depression, allergies, fertility and other issues all depend on the link between our gut and our brain, and the balance of our gut flora.

And yet, too few women make the connection between what they eat (or don't eat) and their health. Unfortunately, neither do their doctors, sometimes! What should you be eating to balance your hormones? This is a big topic and you will get different answers, depending on who you ask. Despite the fact that there are so many diets suggesting that one food choice or the other works for all women, experience shows that **nutritional advice only works if it is tailored to your lifestyle, your culture, your intolerances**, and other parameters.

A raw vegan diet has helped some women resolve severe health issues, whilst other women suddenly perk up when they start re-introducing animal protein and cooked meals.

Some of us eat too much; others don't eat enough. Intermittent fasting, currently very popular and quite beneficial for some women, is not necessarily adequate for those who need to stabilise their blood sugar.

Furthermore, we may eat certain foods for years before noticing that they create inflammation or acidity – this may eventually lead to a severe imbalance.

On a different note, it is not necessarily the meal itself that causes issues, often it is the stressful surroundings in which we eat, or the fact that we don't chew well enough before swallowing our food.

During a consultation, a specialist will listen to you and endeavour to understand your present state in the context of your past habits and of your current lifestyle. If need be, she will ask you to have your blood and stool tested, looking for parasites, heavy metals, information about your gut flora, some inflammation markers, and possible hidden intolerances. Some experts may even proceed to do a genetic test. Ask your family doctor what options you have if going to see a private specialist is not possible.

The natural methods introduced in this book can be a useful complement to your tailor-made dietary recommendations. The link between digestion, stress and hormones is so important and so under-valued, that it deserves a good amount of space in a book about feminine wellbeing. **A healthy belly allows you to face the stress which forms part of life.**

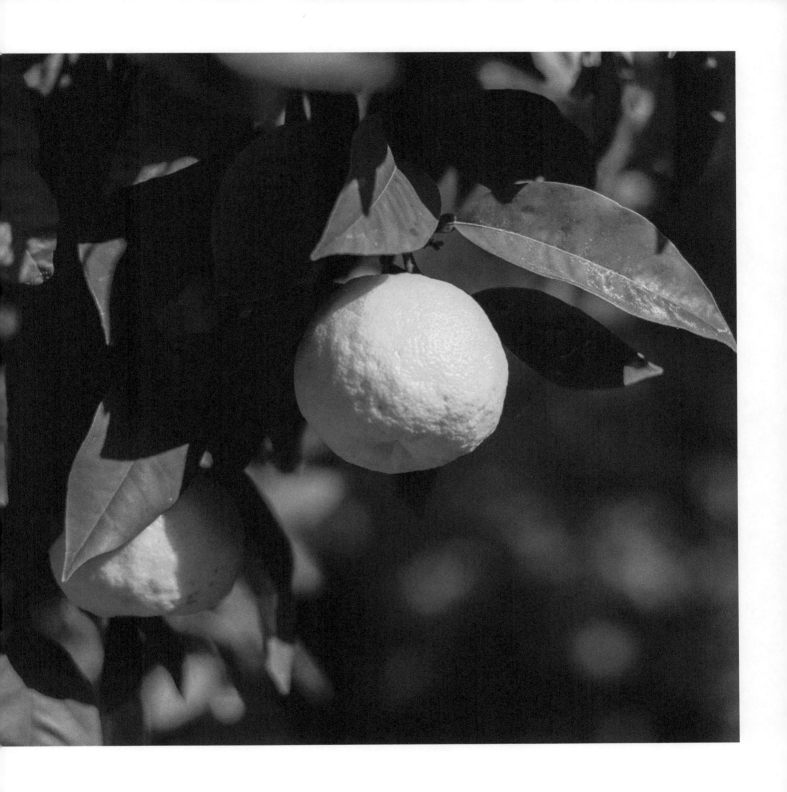

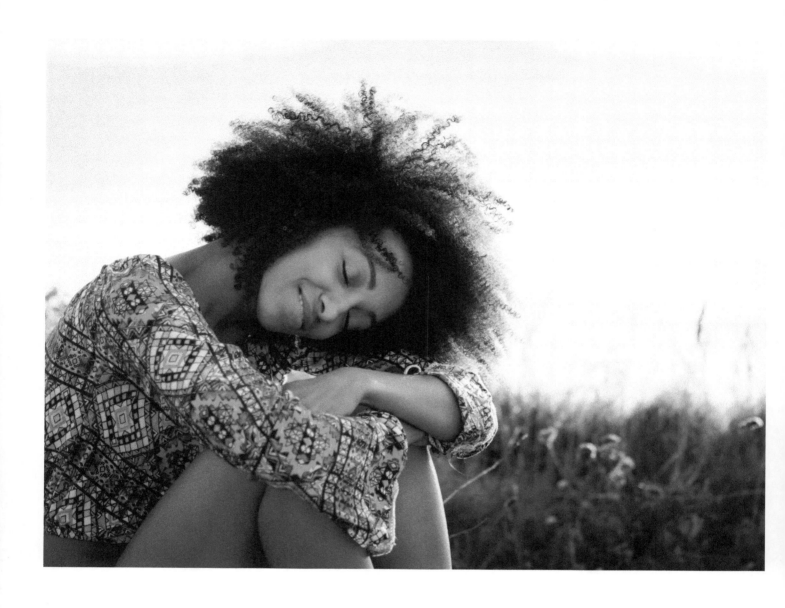

Disconnection

This is not the same as physical rest: **I mean disconnecting form the outside world in order to reconnect with your intuition**. This element is about meditation, in its different expressions, and also simply about **silence, such a rare commodity in our society**. The daily stress may well be of an emotional nature, and quite often we are not even able to pinpoint "what's wrong", because we need to step back in order to see the big picture.

Healing a physical symptom requires factoring in the emotions and the state of mind. Meditation makes us conscious of what is going on, and this is essential in order to implement long-term change. It also helps us to detach, even briefly, from a feeling or a thought that may have become habitual or obsessive. Stepping back is crucial on the path of wellbeing. **Just as our body has an astonishing ability to regenerate, so too our subconscious mind often knows the answer to our most puzzling questions**. Even though meditation is supposed to be undertaken with no specific results in mind, I have noticed time and again that a yoga nidra session, a meditative walk, or sitting for a while with a focus on the breath, can bring crystal-clear answers to complicated situations!

The meditation techniques offered here are very accessible and come from yoga and mindfulness teachings. For those of you who are new to these moments of silence, 3 or 5 minutes may seem long at the beginning, and so many thoughts will race through your mind. First of all: this is normal; it does not mean that you are "no good at this".

Second, **the good news is that we can practise entering into silence in the same way as we practise anything else**, or as we create a new habit. It does become easier, especially if you do the movement and rest sequence first, and if you have not ingested too many stimulants during the day.

A state of inner calm can also be reached through any simple and quiet activity which still requires a certain amount of concentration: handicrafts, calligraphy, gardening, a colouring book, the Japanese tea ceremony, etc.

Meditation is practised both alone and in groups. Some people manage to meditate anywhere, but for most of us, a quiet and clean spot will be more appropriate.

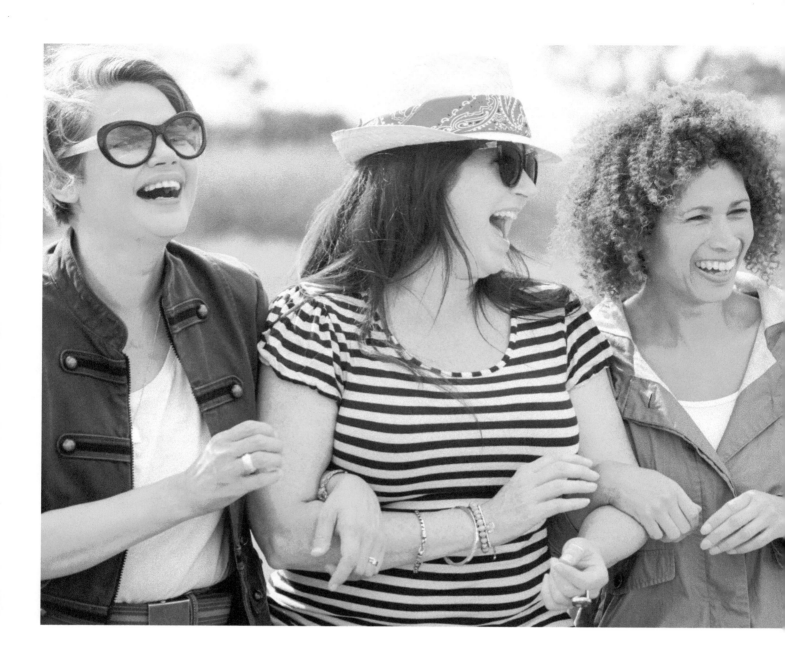

Connection

This element seems to be the opposite of the preceding one, but it really is the other side of the same coin! **The fact that so many individuals live an isolated life, without a "tribe", is not in line with our evolution.** People's personal needs clearly vary in this area, depending on their disposition and their upbringing (those brought up in an environment where they were never alone may seek the same atmosphere, or crave solitude).

Bear in mind also that our chosen "tribe" may be very different from our biological family. What a relief we experience when we meet a group of people who are "on our wave-length", accept us, understand us, support us!

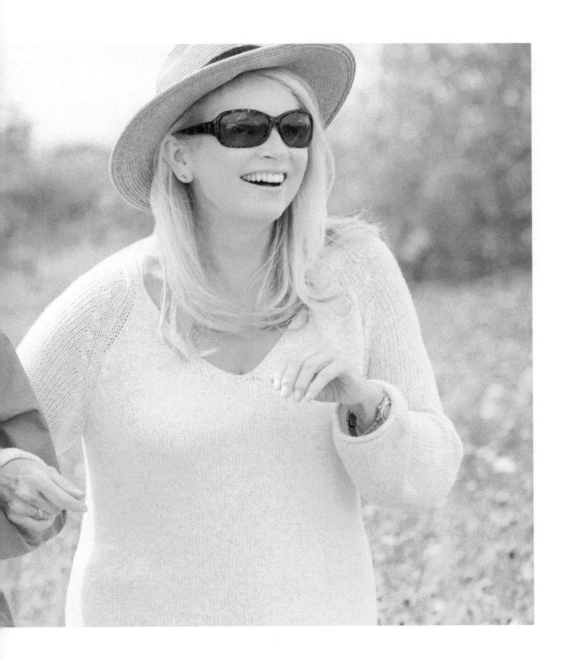

Most of us are no longer subject to the same social or religious rules which applied to our grandmothers and mothers, **we are not condemned to perpetuating their way of life if it does not suit us**. Our life is often very different from the one of the women before us. **On the other hand, the lack of clear markers and rituals creates a feeling of instability and insecurity.** The elders may feel "useless", the younger ones "lost", the ancestral chain of transmission from mother to daughter has been interrupted.

This currently encourages many women to join online chatrooms, be it to exchange ideas with other brides, other young mums or other perimenopausal women, who may well be living in different countries.

These networks are useful and replace, to a certain extent, the knowledge transmission of tribal societies, yet the element of physical presence is missing – **a smile, a tone of voice, a glance, staying together in silence, laughing, feeling strong as a group... such precious moments**. I often notice the benefits of group meetings (as long as they are friendly, of course!) in pre- and postnatal yoga, but also during my yoga workshops on women's issues. This is why I chose to end this book by introducing a special tool: women's circles. **You may then also realise that this book is itself a virtual women's circle**, since you will hear several different voices, and a number of wonderful women came together to co-create it.

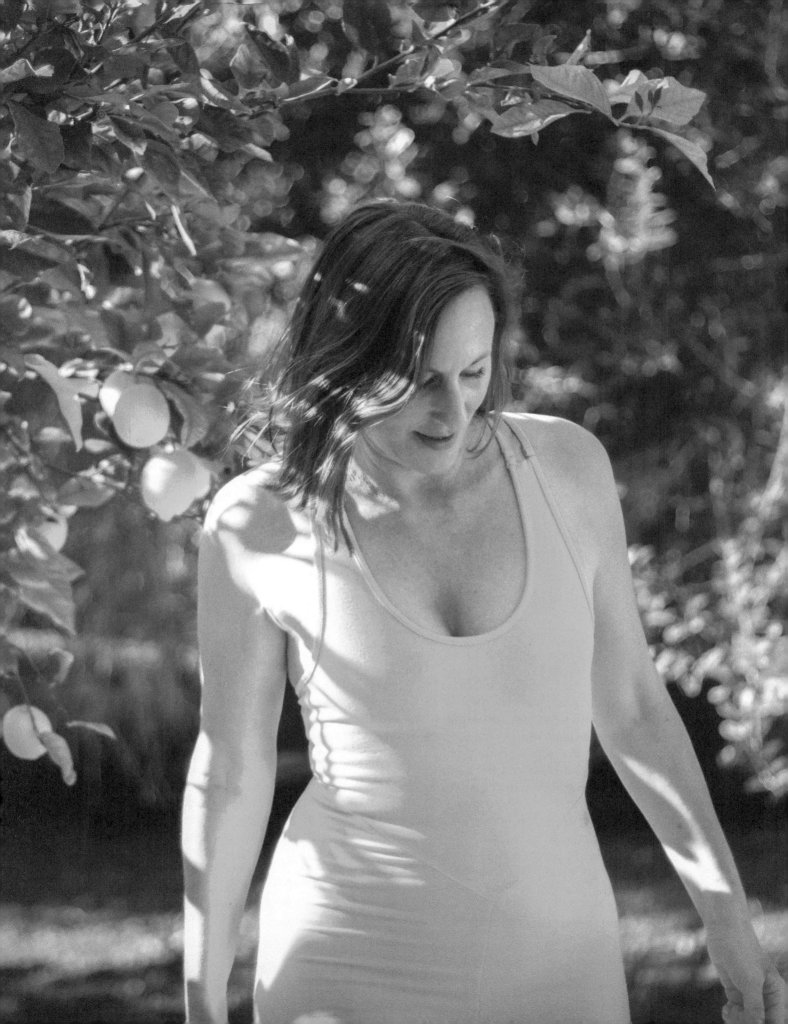

Strength and fragility of the female body

We'll have a look at hormones, organs, nerves and muscles, but your **body is not a machine**, so we will also mention emotions and the environment.
Imbalances will tend to show up first in the most vulnerable part of your body. This vulnerability may be something you were born with, or the result of an accident, an operation or giving birth. It could also be due to external factors such as an improper diet, or exposure to toxic substances.

This book offers no miracle solution, but presents useful information to help you better understand what is going on, and suggests simple ideas to apply in order to improve your daily wellbeing. As we travel down through the body, we'll take a closer look at:

The body's "axes",

managed from our head by the hypothalamus and the pituitary gland, which communicate with the adrenals, the thyroid and the ovaries. These are the "control centres" of the hormonal system and the metabolism: unexplained weight gain or loss, fatigue, hot flushes, heart palpitations, fertility, hypo- and hyperthyroidism - these glands organise everything, and they do so by communicating via hormones and neurotransmitters. These are the pathways in which medication such as the contraceptive pill or antidepressants intervene.

The digestive system.

Digestion is one of the five elements of wellbeing, and it is impossible to be well if this is out of kilter. We will see how the digestive organs regulate not only our elimination, but also our skin, our sleep and our mood. What can we do to support them?

The sexual organs: ovaries, uterus, and vagina. We'll also mention the breasts.

This is where you will find creativity, motherhood, perimenopause, as well as the premenstrual syndrome, period pain, or endometriosis.

The pelvic floor, the vulva and the clitoris.

This very intimate and often unfamiliar area, which will conclude our travels around the female body, will be important for urinary incontinence and, of course, for sexual pleasure.

"It's all in the head" – the body's axes

Our skull contains two tiny areas in the middle of our brain: the **hypothalamus and the pituitary gland**, which oversee a number of systems, also called "axes". In order to keep the female body balanced, three glands - **the adrenals, the thyroid and the ovaries** - constantly exchange messages with these two areas in the head.

The messengers transmitting this information between the head and the organs in order to maintain balance (= homeostasis) are the **hormones** (for the endocrine system) and the **neurotransmitters** (for the nervous system).

The hypothalamus is an organ which regulates hunger and thirst, waking and sleeping, and most of the body's involuntary ("automatic") mechanisms.

It sends signals to the pituitary gland, just below, an endocrine gland which influences **growth, metabolism and regeneration**.

The varying levels of hormones from the adrenals, the thyroid, and the ovaries send messages in return, which is called *feedback*. This loop protects the organism against excessively high or low levels of hormones.

The three axes

Science distinguishes between 3 axes, but you will soon understand that they are not strictly separate. In fact, **the adrenals, the ovaries, and the thyroid interact, and their functions also overlap**.

The hormonal system could be compared with an orchestra – all instruments must play in sync to create a harmonious melody.

Therefore, when you receive a diagnosis which mentions one of the axes, if you take medication which targets one of them, or if you have certain genetic predispositions, remember to also take the other two "loops" into consideration.

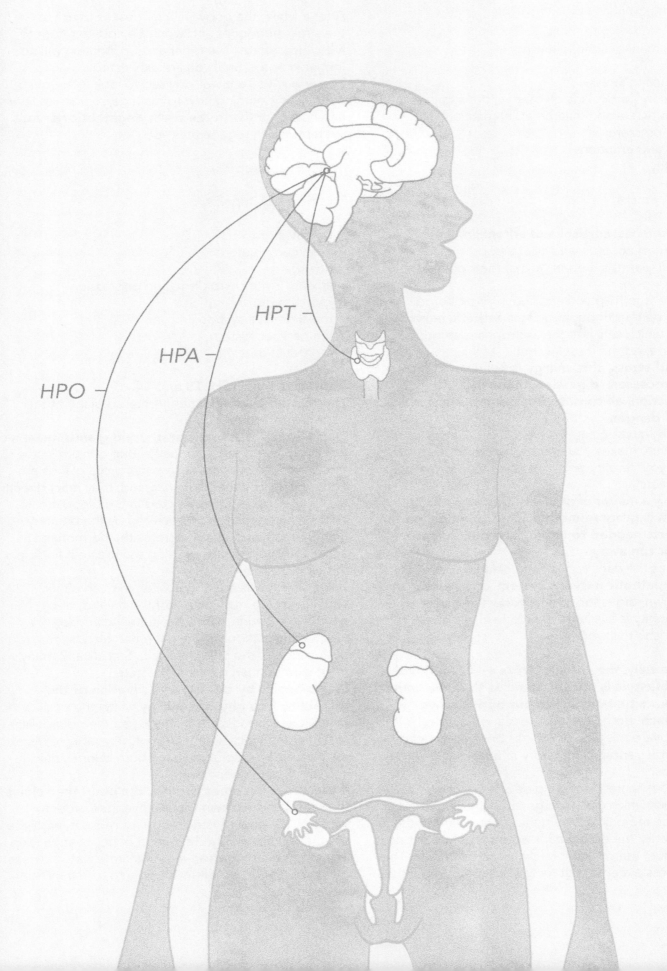

This axis manages the following:

- reactions to stress
- digestion (particularly glycaemia, the sugar level)
- immunity (the anti-inflammatory reaction)
- blood pressure
- mood and emotions
- sexuality
- bones
- energy stocks.

Main hormones: **cortisol and adrenalin**, the hormones of action… and of stress, produced by two small glands sitting on top of the kidneys, the adrenals.
Their role is to help you act, and in particular to face any danger through the **sympathetic nervous system**, which sets free the appropriate amount of energy to feed the muscles, brain, and heart.
In case of stress, this energy is "diverted" from other processes: digestion, immunity and reproduction, all considered less important in times of danger.
This is why stress creates digestive issues, causes weight gain, makes you more sensitive to infections, impacts your fertility, and lowers your libido (amongst other effects).
It is simply a matter of priorities: **the stressed organism is programmed to focus primarily on the body parts needed to either face the danger and fight – or run away**.
As soon as the danger has been cleared, the **parasympathetic nervous system** kicks in: everything calms down, digestion and reproduction can resume, and immunity is available to help heal any fresh wounds. Isn't this wonderful?

Unfortunately, the chronic stress associated with today's lifestyle is not the same as the time-limited dangerous situations which our body knows how to face. Both "social" stress and "physical" stress activate this axis, which has been associated with allergies and inflammatory or auto-immune conditions.[iii]
The wolf we feared in the old days is now an alarm clock which always rings too early, an unkind supervisor, the delayed train that gets us late to the school gates, the empty bank account before the next pay cheque, the constant background noise, etc. This stress is less extreme, but more constant or repetitive.

After a while, the body will be "desensitised" to the stress hormones and won't be able to return to a balanced state. The regeneration function will no longer kick in… until you are exhausted.
This is why you are well advised to look after your adrenals by learning how to manage your stress levels and how to **activate the parasympathetic nervous system**, which regenerates you.

This pathway impacts:

- body weight
- body temperature
- heartbeat
- anxiety (hyperthyroidism) and depression (hypothyroidism)
- the digestive system
- the nervous system
- reproduction.

Main hormones: **TSH, T3 and T4.**
The thyroid is a tiny butterfly-shaped gland at the base of the throat.
On its two sides are the **parathyroid glands** (there are usually 4), which regulate the level of calcium in the blood and the bones. Those parathyroid glands are not managed by the pituitary gland; they react directly to the level of calcium detected in the bloodstream.
When it receives the TSH secreted by the pituitary gland, the thyroid gland secretes the hormones T3 and T4, and it does so by using the iodine it finds in the bloodstream.
When TSH levels are out of kilter, this can either be caused by a malfunction of the thyroid, or by a problem coming from the pituitary gland (a miscommunication between the two glands, or a dysfunction of the pituitary itself). Statistically, many more women than men are affected.
Stress begins by causing an activation of the thyroid to free physical energy which the body thinks it needs to face the danger, so the metabolism accelerates. Typically, a person with hyperthyroidism will have heart palpitations, will burn calories quickly, and suffer from sleep issues.
If the stress becomes chronic, the body then slows the metabolism down via the thyroid in order to switch to "energy saving" mode, because it reads the situation as a prolonged situation of deprivation (akin to a long trek through an area with little water). Those with hypothyroidism often struggle to lose their extra

weight, may often shiver and feel cold, and even move more slowly.

This shows that stress, which is mainly managed by the adrenals, also directly affects the thyroid. As a result, when our adrenals are "depleted", a medical treatment of the thyroid gland may not be well tolerated, which is why functional medicine specialists generally advise treating the adrenals first.

When checking blood work for thyroid imbalances, some doctors only measure the TSH, yet many nowadays also insist on checking the levels of T3 and T4, as well as looking for specific antibodies (Anti-thyroid peroxidase or 'anti-TPO' antibodies), which would indicate an auto-immune condition: Hashimoto's for hypothyroidism, Graves or Basedow for hyperthyroidism. These conditions appear when the immune system attacks the thyroid gland, and they are increasingly frequent.

Specialists' opinions differ when it comes to defining a "normal level" of TSH. Functional medicine and naturopaths, but also some specialists of degenerative diseases such as Dr Dale Bredesen, consider a TSH level below 2 uUI/ml as optimal, whereas the British Thyroid Foundation points out that laboratories set a wider reference range for TSH: between 0.4 and 4.0.
The higher the number, the more sluggish the thyroid is considered to be. Therefore, your doctor may say you are "still in the normal range", although you don't feel well.

Puberty, pregnancy and menopause, the three big hormonal shifts in a woman's life, **often impact the thyroid**, because it reacts to the level of oestrogens in the bloodstream: they lower or heighten the absorption levels of iodine by the gland. This imbalance, caused by the modification of the ovaries' activity, can be temporary, and does not always require life-long medication.
There is also a verified (although not quite understood) link between polycystic ovary syndrome (PCOS) and thyroid auto-immune conditions .
Furthermore, another crucial interaction is often ignored: the link between thyroid and digestion.
Amongst other things, the thyroid needs iodine, selenium, iron and magnesium in order to function well. Even if your meals contained enough of them (which is often not the case, due to depleted topsoil, long journeys, and industrial transformation of foods), a lack of absorption at the digestive level because of food intolerances or an imbalance in the gut flora can cause thyroid issues.

"Hypothalamic-Pituitary-Ovarian (HPO) axis".

This axis manages:

o development and regulation of the reproductive system: uterus, ovaries and secondary sexual characteristics (mainly breasts, pubic hair, hips)
o bones
o immune system
o ageing of tissues.

Main hormones: **LH and FSH, oestrogens** (mainly oestradiol, oestriol and oestrone) **and testosterone**, in short: the sexual hormones.
FSH and LH are secreted by the pituitary gland and stimulate the production of oestrogen and inhibin by the ovaries, which regulates the menstrual cycle.
During puberty, the HPO axis is activated when the ovaries secrete oestrogens. This causes the physiological and psychological transformation of adolescents, both male and female. In men, this axis (connected to the testes instead of the ovaries) once activated, stays more or less active over the person's lifetime (in principle at least), but **in women, another significant change on this axis will induce menopause**.
In women of childbearing age, the feedback between oestrogens and LH prepares the ovarian follicle for ovulation, and the uterus for the possible implantation of a fertilised egg. After ovulation, the empty follicle produces progesterone, which interrupts the oestrogen-LH loop and makes sure that a period does not occur if the egg has been fertilised. The placenta then takes over and keeps producing progesterone; the mother-to-be will therefore not ovulate again until after she has given birth. If no egg has been fertilised, progesterone secretion will dwindle, menstruation will happen, and the cycle of oestrogen production starts again.

The HPA axis interacts in several ways with the ovarian axis: as we saw, it can block fertility in the case of stress. Again, the body means well: better not to be pregnant in a dangerous or unstable situation.
The adrenals also produce a small quantity of oestrogens, which helps to soften the hormonal transition of menopause. And yet another body part produces oestrogens: the adipose tissue, aka fat, especially in the belly area.
Jani White, whom you will meet in this book, says that throughout perimenopause, the body makes

sure to stock oestrogen in the body fat around the hips. By dieting to eliminate this fatty tissue, we deprive the body of oestrogens which it wants to use in order to ensure a healthy menopause. Yet as always, balance is key here: too much body fat can often explain an excess of oestrogens and the ensuing problems, which we will mention later.

The contraceptive pill works on the HPO axis, by interrupting the loop, so that the follicle does not develop and there is no ovulation.

Suppressing ovulation is also used to prepare for **in vitro fertilisation treatment**, in order to better control the time to harvest the eggs. This is also where intervention happens to suppress oestrogen production in cases of hormone-related cancers. Finally, **Hormone Replacement Therapy (HRT)** for women in perimenopause also intervenes on this axis, by adding oestrogens and progesterone which the ovaries are no longer producing.

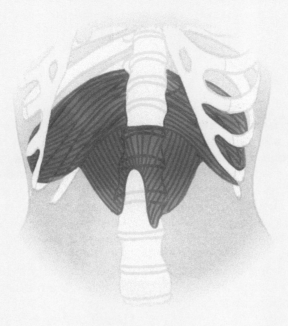

The **diaphragm** is a form of birth control, right? Well, yes, but also a large muscle in your body: a kind of parachute or dome which separates the belly from the chest. When it sinks down, it makes more space for your lungs, which are like two bags. They fill with air: that's an inhalation. By lifting up again, the diaphragm "pushes upwards" against the bottom of the lungs and the air is automatically expelled via the nostrils: that's an exhalation.

By breathing more slowly and deeply, we send a signal to the brain: all is well, the body is relaxed, you can now activate the **parasympathetic nervous system**. When we are stressed, our breathing pattern is quicker and more superficial (sometimes to the point of hyperventilation). To calm your nervous system, try focusing on long exhalations. Example: inhale to a count of 3 and exhale to a count of 4 or 5, or even more. Always do what is comfortable and never strain the breath.

NB: if you are suffering with depression this practice is not recommended as extending the exhalation often becomes more of a "sigh", and this is not helpful when depressed. Instead focus on an easy and steady rhythm of breath, with the inhale and exhale of equal length.

In any case, this isn't about forcing anything. Rather try to imagine the breath like a wave, which comes in to the shore and retreats again. You may also enjoy adding a soft sound to your breath by slightly "closing" the front of your throat so the breath moves more through the back of the throat, creating an ocean-like sound. This is called "**Ujjayi**" breath in yoga, and you could also think of it as being like the sound of the wind in the trees. Again, always be careful to never strain when trying this breath.

Place your hands on your lowest ribs. Feel how the ribs expand sideways on the inhalation, away from your centre, and then come closer again on the exhalation. Unlike what you may sometimes hear teachers say, do not push out your belly like a balloon on the inhalation, rather allow it to soften naturally. On the exhalation, gently engage your abdominal muscles and feel the navel drawing inwards and slightly upwards, towards the ribs.
There you go! This is your secret weapon to face a challenging situation.

This thin fibrous membrane creates a network throughout the human body, a bit like an actual net which would maintain a desired shape. If you observe a piece of raw meat, you will notice a delicate white membrane around the flesh and, especially in the case of red meat, denser and thicker fibres running through it – this is exactly what we are talking about.

Fascia can be thicker or thinner, depending on their location. They are built, among other things, from collagen and elastin – no wonder we often find these words in the list of ingredients for anti-ageing creams.

Visceral fascia is the least extensible, it covers the organs to keep them in place and avoid a prolapse, meaning organs sinking down due to the effect of gravity.

These membranes retract in case of trauma, repeated postural imbalances, lack of physical activity, dehydration, stress… This will feel as if you are stuck in a tight wetsuit, in which you can hardly move. It causes restriction of your range of movement.

Meridians, these energy channels of the Chinese tradition, as well *nadis*, their equivalent in Ayurveda, are situated in what we call fascia today.

Western science has only recently developed an interest in fascia, which used to simply be discarded during anatomical dissections. We are beginning to understand that these membranes are more than a structure; they form a communication network through which messages are exchanged. This helps to explain why hormonal signals seem to be hindered by a very stiff body, and also why an imbalance in one part of the body can manifest elsewhere, which is something to bear in mind when assessing your feminine health issues.

Women's hormones actually have an effect upon the fascia: fluctuations in the levels of oestrogens and relaxin (especially during ovulation, menstruation and pregnancy), influence collagen production. The body can therefore feel more flexible, but also less stable, which explains why problems with ankles, knees, hips, wrists, and shoulders are more frequent at those times.

"Use it or lose it" – **If you don't move your body regularly and in a variety of ways, it will become stiffer**, because fascia are hydrated by a combination of movement, fluid intake (drink good quality water!) and rest. Too much movement without adequate rest does not give the fascia time to rehydrate and will create tension, hence more potential injuries.

There are people who specialise in treating fascia through touch: Myofascial Release Therapy is a form of therapeutic massage which helps give these tissues more elasticity, with impressive results.

You can also improve your range of movement by working on the fascia through slow and conscious movement practises such as yoga, particularly yin yoga, which specialises in this. Holding a posture for a long time, going into a deep stretch without first warming up the muscle, will work on the fascia. You'll want to avoid damaging the tissues with excessive or wrongly placed effort, so it is worth learning yin yoga with a qualified instructor (such as Mirjam Wagner from our women's circle). Tai chi and qigong, as well as other Chinese martial arts, also target the fascia.

Endocrine disruptors

Apart from the effects of **stress** we explained above, women are slowly becoming more mindful of the fact that they are surrounded, in their everyday lives, by substances which interrupt the optimal functioning of the three axes, namely **endocrine disruptors**.

This is how the World Health Organisation defined them in 2002: "*an exogenous substance or mixture that alters function(s) of the endocrine system and consequently causes adverse health effects in an intact organism, or its progeny, or (sub)populations*".[iv]

Endocrine disruptors can be of natural origin (hormones and phytoestrogens) or result from human activities. They can be contained in common consumer goods, in agricultural chemicals, in prescription drugs or cosmetics. The 2012 WHO-UNEP report lists approximately 800 chemical substances with proven or suspected endocrine disrupting effects. The list is regularly updated. Among them:
◦ some pesticides (organochlorines, fungicides, herbicides)
◦ plasticisers (phthalates, Bisphenol A), flame retardants (BDE), liners (PFAs)
◦ drugs: Diethylstilboestrol, painkillers (paracetamol), antidepressants (fluoxetine)
◦ incinerators and transformers (dioxins, furans, PCB)
◦ some hygiene products, such as Triclosan
◦ phytoestrogens such as soy.

We are exposed to them in various ways (swallowing, inhalation, skin contact), and mostly in low doses. **A massive or repeated exposure to these substances can create a problem with something that would, in principle, be manageable by the body in small quantities.**

Endocrine disruptors will mimic the action of a natural hormone and trigger a reaction that corresponds to this hormone, or in contrast block a hormone from docking to its receptor and stop the transmission of the hormonal signal. They can also disrupt the production or regulation of the hormones themselves, or of their receptors. **These substances can modify several processes, such as the regulation of metabolism and development**; they notably risk disrupting the entire reproduction cycle, from fertility to the development of the foetus during pregnancy.

How to destress and go into "rest and recharge" mode?

◦ At the physical level, learn how to **activate the parasympathetic nervous system** by moving the lumbar and cervical part of the spine (see our yoga session), by practising slow and deep breathing (see our tip) and by taking short breaks throughout your day, preferably outside, in nature.
◦ Choose cosmetics, cleaning products, clothes, furniture and food without **endocrine disruptors** where possible, and add potted plants to closed spaces, to filter the air.
◦ Improve your **digestion** and buy good quality foods, so your glands receive the nourishment they need.
◦ Create situations which help you to secrete **oxytocin**, a hormone produced during pleasant social interactions and massages, and which calms the three axes, helping you manage your stress (see the chapter on women's circles).

Acupuncture, Homeopathy, and Ayurveda: listening to your body

What is the big advantage of "alternative" therapies, compared to prescription drug hormone therapy? Very little side effects, so that you can avoid creating another problem whilst fixing a first issue. Furthermore, their approach is holistic, since they aim to rebalance the entire organism and to understand which external factors contributed to the imbalance in the first place.
NB: The experts which provided the texts below asked me to point out that these healing systems each have their own history and internal logic. Even though some elements might overlap, it is recommended, if you feel like trying them, to choose one and stick with it long enough to give it a chance to work, rather than switching between them or mixing them.

HOW ACUPUNCTURE CAN HELP

by Jani White

Acupuncture is one component of Traditional Chinese Medicine (TCM), which is a Whole Systems Medicine in its own right. TCM uses its own unique language to describe the way that our human bodies function. This is a different language than we use in Western Allopathic medicine, BUT, we are looking at the same physiology, the same psychology, the same effects of pathology.

Chinese medicine as a whole encompasses acupuncture, herbs, moxibustion, cupping, *gua sha* (body work), *tui na* (massage), and most importantly, diet and lifestyle advice according to your constitutional diagnosis.

In Chinese medicine we are able to diagnose the 'type' of constitution you have, and to particularly tailor the treatment to meet the specific needs of YOUR body, YOUR emotional circumstances, and to look particularly at the interplay between YOUR emotional and physical self. It is a highly tailored medicine that is able to look at the unique circumstances that add up to your particular experience; taking into account the physical symptoms you are experiencing in the context of the emotional circumstances you are experiencing.

We are humans. Our physiology is completely entwined with our psychology. We are one massive bundle of experience.

Acupuncture, perhaps the most well-known aspect of Chinese medicine is all about the systems of communication in your body. Perhaps you have heard about the idea of the meridian, or channel systems...

One of the best ways to describe this is to think of the Paris Metro or the London Underground. You know you need to get from A to B. There is a whole system of 'lines' (channels) that allow you to travel from one part of the city to another. You can look at the map, and you can decide how to travel along one line, then transfer at a certain place to access another, and so on, until you are able to reach your destination in the most efficient way possible.

Along the acupuncture channels there are a series of 'points', the places where we insert the acupuncture needles. Think of that Metro line. You enter the station at ground level - inserting the needle into the point - and we drop deep into that underground system of intersecting lines. By sequencing a series of needles into various acupuncture points we are able to create a connection of communication that gets us from A to B.

Acupuncture is ALL about hormones. Our bodies work via an astonishing network of over 100 trillion neurons (yes, that is the number!) triggering (synapsing) the vast amount of communications it takes your body to function. These trillions of neurons are triggering your hormones to do the things they do to keep us functioning in good health.

The governance of our physiologic responses are hormonally triggered. The way that our body determines how to keep its balance is to ensure that everything happens in the correct sequence. This is governed by what are called 'feedback loops'. Certain hormones are triggered, activating certain responses, which when resolved send further hormone 'feedback' to regulate the balance and switch on or off the hormone flows that dictate what should happen.

When we experience ANY of the negative symptoms that we associate with female health disruption - irregular or uncomfortable periods, PCOS, endometriosis, menopausal symptoms, infertility, every disruptive aspect of pregnancy birth and recovery - ALL of these irregularities suggest a breakdown in the feedback loops that regulate our hormones.

Our female health is predicated on the smooth communication of our HPO - the Hypothalamus Pituitary Ovarian Axis - which governs the smooth flow and sequencing of our sexual and reproductive hormones.

We, as females, as humans, are also subject to the feedback regulation of the HPA - the Hypothalamus Pituitary Adrenal Axis - which governs our stress response.

These feedback loops, the HPO and HPA are the principal governance of our gynaecological and emotional responses.

So let's go back to thinking about that analogy of the Metro and the idea of the channels that allow us to map the intersection of these lines of communication. And now let's add another level of analogy to that. So the acupuncture needles have gone into certain points to sequence together a pathway of communication…

Now let's add the idea of how we use our mouse when we are working on our computer. We can move our mouse in any direction, and we can ask it to add information, or delete it, or move something from one file to another, or we can merge things or create a master file, or separate a conglomerate into separate files…

With our mouse we have the ability to dictate how we wish the information to be used in order to affect a response. The way we use the acupuncture needles, how we manipulate the needles once they are inserted, is like managing the mouse. Our subtle movements with the needles help to determine how the flow of information is being dictated.

This is how acupuncture works. We are able, through the very holistic Chinese medical diagnosis, to determine the correlations in your body's response to the environmental and emotional influences that are affecting you. Through careful deduction, we can understand which acupoints to use to help to regulate the flow of the HPO and HPA, and coordinate the needles to help influence those trillions of synapses to regulate your function.

Acupuncture seems to be somewhat magical, but that is only because of the extraordinary capacity of your human physiology. Acupuncture affects the communication of those trillions of synapses - the triggers of communication that tell your hormones what to do - and helps to influence those hormone feedback loops to do what they do best - to regulate.

Though it seems magical, in reality acupuncture is entirely neurobiological. It truly is a marvellous way for us to balance our hormones by activating our body's own hormone regulation tools.

Voilà!

HOMEOPATHY AND WOMEN'S HORMONES

by Sarah Davison

For many people, homeopathy is a bit of a mystery. They know it's natural, but not much more than that. So let's start by demystifying it, and making clear what it is, and what it isn't.

Homeopathy is...

○ a system of medicine that uses a nano-dose of the substance, that if you overdosed on it, would cause symptoms similar to those you have. In this way, it stimulates your innate self-healing system to resolve the problem..

○ the second most popular system of medicine in the world after conventional medicine with, according to the World Health Organisation, an estimated 450 million users.

○ 100% natural, with no side-effects.

○ focused on treating the whole person, not just the isolated symptoms, thereby honouring the link between mind and body, and the interconnectedness of the body's different systems.

○ used to treat the whole spectrum of illness from minor to chronic, and from physical and mental, to emotional and spiritual.

○ supported by scientific evidence. There is a small, but robust body of scientific evidence showing it is more than placebo (www.hri-research.org).

○ safe to use alongside, or to withdraw from, conventional medicines, though the latter should involve the supervision of the physician who prescribed the medicine.

Homeopathy is not...

○ nutritional supplements or herbs, though the latter are the source material for many homeopathic medicines.

○ dietary or lifestyle advice, although these things may form a small part of homeopathic treatment.

How homeopathy is different from conventional medicine

Homeopaths see symptoms as what the body or mind creates in order to heal itself e.g. a fever is designed to burn off an infection. So in an acute illness like flu for instance, a homeopathic remedy will serve to speed up the healing process. Whereas in a chronic illness, (which is when the self-healing mechanism has got stuck repeating the same symptoms without a healing resolution), homeopathy stimulates that mechanism to complete the process of healing.

Homeopathy for women's wellness

When it comes to women's wellness, as with any other area of health, a homeopath will not only be looking at the whole person - body, mind and emotion - but also for potential underlying causes that need to be addressed in order to ensure an effective, lasting cure. Here are some examples of causes within the arena of women's health:

○ a hormonal shift e.g. puberty, childbirth or menopause.

○ a bad reaction to a medical drug e.g. the contraceptive pill, HRT, an anti-depressant.

○ a sluggish liver or gut which, due to diet, suppressed anger, medications, low thyroid etc, cannot rid the body of excess hormones.

○ an anxious personality, who is chronically stressed, leading to disturbed hormonal balance.

○ a woman who finds it difficult to say no to others, and struggles to look after her own needs - causing stress, suppressed anger, which links to the above two points.

Looking at menopause specifically, many women feel they face an impossible choice between suffering and flooding their bodies with synthetic hormones. Homeopathy is one answer to this dilemma, as you can see from the case stories below. In addition, there is scientific evidence to support its effectiveness: In an observational study of 438 women across eight countries, 99% reported the disappearance or reduction of their hot flushes - the majority within 15 days of starting homeopathic treatment. And a randomised, controlled trial with 133 women suffering menopausal depression, compared homeopathy, the anti-depressant fluoxetine, and placebo. Results showed homeopathy and fluoxetine to be equally effective in reducing depression. However, the difference was that homeopathy also resolved a number of other menopause symptoms such as hot flushes.

Stories of women's wellness helped by homeopathy
These stories are mostly of women aged 35-65 with difficulties triggered by menopause. But the symptoms described do not just occur in menopause.

Vaginal dryness
L's vaginal dryness started in menopause and got steadily worse. Aged 59, she experienced intense burning during intercourse, which had not responded to the conventional oestradiol vaginal tablets. After only one month of homeopathy, she reported being 90% better.

Hot flushes
At 50, A's periods had started to become irregular, and as part of her peri-menopause, she was also experiencing hot flushes. Within a few months on homeopathic remedies, her hot flushes were a thing of the past.

Tearfulness, menstrual flooding & dry skin
At 46, M's periods were irregular, prolonged and extremely heavy. She also had very dry skin, and was becoming unusually tearful under stress. Within three months of starting treatment, her periods had normalised, her skin had improved, and she was calm under stress.

Anxiety, irritability, PMS, joint pain
After two months on homeopathy, C, aged 44, noticed great improvements in her anxiety, extreme irritability (especially before her period), low mood, joint pain, disturbed sleep, and hot flushes.

Ovulation & PMS problems
Here is a text I received from H., 45: "No problems with ovulation or PMS this cycle!!! As PMS was about to hit, I was dreading it and then as the days passed and I had neither nausea, nor headache, nor over the top emotivity, nor sleepless nights, I was happily puzzled! What a relief…Thank you a thousand times!"

Treat yourself or see a homeopath?
In some countries you can buy homeopathic combinations and single remedies for minor illnesses like flu, insomnia, headaches etc., at the pharmacy. This is wonderful, because it gives the public easy access to the amazing power of homeopathy. And in many cases, that is all that is needed. However, self-treatment has its downsides:
○ Some who have had success with a self-prescribed remedy continue to take it once better, and then find they get worse again. This is because they are unaware that taking too much of a remedy you no longer need, can cause the symptoms you have just cured.
○ Others have no success with the chosen remedy, because it is not the best match for their symptoms. For every symptom there are tens, often hundreds, of possible homeopathic remedies, e.g. for menstrual pain there are 468 remedies. So the process of finding the most effective remedy can be complex, and is best done by a professional homeopath.
In summary, homeopathy is a natural, gentle and effective form of medicine particularly well-suited to helping women navigate hormonal challenges.

REGAIN HEALTH AND VITALITY WITH AYURVEDA

by Stéfanie Lolivret

Amongst the approaches which can complement, or provide an alternative to, modern medicine in order to enhance wellness in women's lives, Ayurveda is one of the key players. Really? Indeed! **Let's have a look at why Ayurveda is so relevant in today's world, and let us put a few of its secrets into practice**.

Ayurveda is a holistic medical system, born in India over 5000 years ago, today recognised by the World Health Organisation. It shares the same origins as yoga. Ayurveda is a Sanskrit word literally translated as "science of life". The term "science" is understood here as understanding and experimenting, rather than a purely intellectual scientific approach. **Ayurveda is above all tangible and pragmatic**. The word "ayur" (life) encompasses the entire phenomenality of living, which includes movement (vayu or prana) and therefore all changes which occur throughout life. And there are plenty of such changes in a woman's life: the big milestones (puberty, motherhood, menopause) and the rhythm of menstrual cycles (ovulation and menstruation) with its plethora of hormonal changes… It is noteworthy, in this context, **that amongst the eight branches of Ayurveda, and at the same level as internal medicine, psychology, or surgery, one branch is entirely dedicated to women and fertility**.

Ayurveda's special feature is first and foremost that it looks at the person, and not just at the illness. The woman is therefore fully honoured as a unique individual. Moreover, she is a being who possesses the divine creative power of giving life. The ayurvedic approach will accompany her throughout her life to allow her to maximise her wellbeing at the physical, mental, energetic, and emotional level. Indeed,

Ayurveda's second special feature is its holistic approach. It addresses the woman at every level of her being, body-mind-consciousness, instead of pursuing a mechanical approach to the physical and biochemical organism. Therefore, everything is connected, and healing a hormonal imbalance can re-establish harmony at the emotional level (and the other way round).

The third specific feature of Ayurveda is that it always seeks to return to the root of the imbalance. A symptom allows us to identify that something is out of kilter, and Ayurveda aims to understand where this began, to identify the energetic imbalance which happened first, in order to intervene over the long term, preventatively and durably.

Consulting an ayurvedic therapist can therefore be a bit disconcerting at first. In order to establish an ayurvedic diagnosis, they will observe your tongue, your nails, your eyes, your pulse, and ask you all sorts of questions which don't seem to be related to your symptom, but rather to your metabolism, your energy … and for good reason: ayurvedic physiology is very different from modern medicine. **According to Ayurveda, the body is first and foremost made of energy, and composed of three fundamental energies (or humours, called *doshas*): *Vata* (air), *Pitta* (fire), and *Kapha* (water)**. These energies exist in all of us in unique proportions, and their mix defines us as individuals. **Influenced by our surroundings, our lifestyle and our** eating habits, this balance is perpetually brought out of kilter and realigns itself, continuously, in a dynamic way. But if the imbalance persists, illness can develop, and its first symptoms will appear. Ayurveda analyses this doshic imbalance and aims to recreate a person's integral harmony.

When it comes to therapeutic advice, be prepared for much more than just swallowing a pill "made in India", because you will be asked to **take an active role in your self-healing by receiving the keys to restoring lasting happiness**. While **Ayurveda offers a plethora of hygiene and lifestyle advice specifically chosen for your constitution** (including massage, yogic techniques… and more!), it is likely that, before tailor-made remedies aimed at your doshic imbalance are offered, **your journey towards increased wellbeing will start by detoxification and regulating your digestion… indeed, nutrition is one of Ayurveda's three pillars**. The first question you will be asked is not "are you eating the right foods?" but rather "is your digestion optimal for transforming and assimilating the nutrients you are ingesting?". An often-neglected aspect of modern medicine is essential in Ayurveda: **digestion is at the heart of your "energetic rebalancing"**. You must be able to fully digest and transform food, to assimilate nutrients, and to eliminate metabolic waste products, in order to be considered healthy from the Ayurvedic point of view. Only then, through balancing the doshas *Vata* (energy of movement), *Pitta* (energy of transformation) and *Kapha* (energy of cohesion), together with the digestive fire of *Agni*, can the tissues (the 7 *dhatus*) be properly formed. Moreover, **you will minimise the formation of toxins (*ama*), the main cause of illness**.

So: take care to optimise your digestion! How? **Eat at the same times every day, preferring cooked and warm meals, based on fresh and natural ingredients, integrating the six ayurvedic flavours** (sweet, acidic, salty, hot, bitter, astringent). **Enjoy your experience by cooking with spices and herbs** to enhance flavours and stimulate your digestive fire. **Savour your meals mindfully**, in a calm atmosphere, engaging all your senses. Your entire being (physical, mental, emotional…) will feel better and you will discover a different taste for Life itself. **A famous Indian saying sums it up well: "Look after your body, so your soul will wish to dwell in it."**

Yoga sequence
focusing on the axes

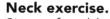

Neck exercise.
Sit comfortably, spine upright, head straight, breathe deeply whilst partly closing your throat (glottis), creating a soft, ocean-like sound (*Ujayyi* **breath**). Keep breathing this way, then on an exhalation turn your head to the right and lower your chin towards the side of your throat. Inhale as you come back to centre, head straight, then exhale to your left, again lowering the chin to the throat. Repeat 6 times on each side.

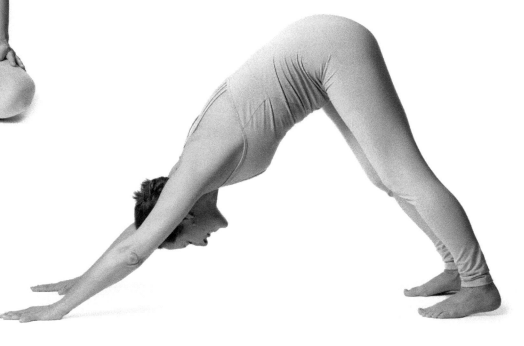

Downward-facing dog.
Come to all fours, hands under your shoulders or slightly further forward if that suits you better, fingers spread and pointing forwards, knees hip distance apart. As you exhale, lift both knees off the ground.

Your hips go up and back at the same time. Keep your knees slightly bent to allow your spine to lengthen up and back. You may wish to lift one heel, then the other, to walk on the spot and stretch your calf muscles, then steady your posture.

No need to touch your heels to the floor at all costs. Keep your ears between your arms. Imagine pushing the floor away with your hands, breathe deeply. When your arms get tired, return to all fours by lowering your knees.

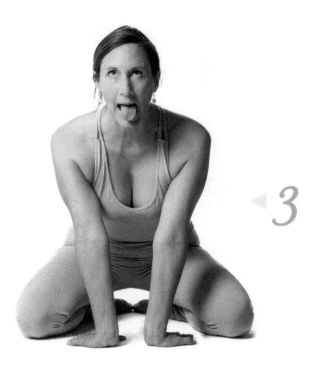

Lion.

Sitting on the floor, with your buttocks on your heels or a pillow, bring your hands to the floor with fingers pointing towards you, if your wrists allow this, or place the hands on your knees, fingers pointing down. Look up to the space between your eyebrows (you'll go a bit cross-eyed). Inhale deeply through the nose, then exhale through the mouth as you stick your tongue out and roar "Haaaaa!". Repeat three times in total

3

Half Shoulder Stand (*avoid during menstruation*).

X! Lie on the floor with a firm but comfortable support under your buttocks. Choose a folded blanket, firm cushions, or a bolster. Lift your legs, knees bent, then unfold your legs, heels towards the ceiling. If a wall is available, rest your legs against the wall. Otherwise just hold them up in the air for as long as you can without straining.

You may wish to stay several minutes. To come out, if you are against the wall, push your feet into the wall to lift your hips, so you can remove the support prop, then pivot on to your right side and stay there for several breaths before sitting up. Without a wall: bend your knees, put the feet on the floor, lift your hips to remove the support and pivot on to your right side before slowly sitting up.

4

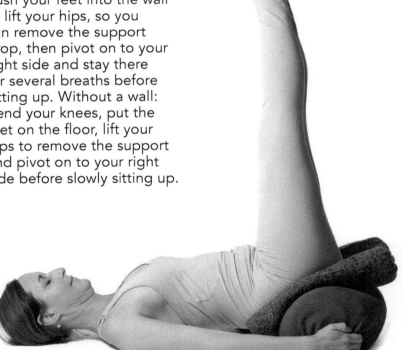

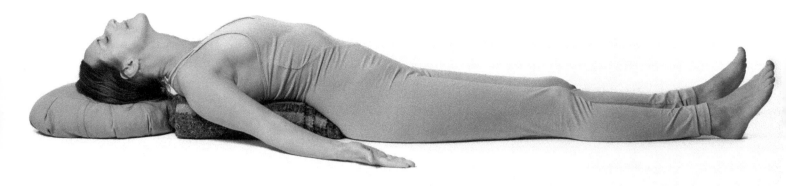

Supported fish (*in pregnancy: OK until week 30, but with a low prop to avoid bending back too deeply*).
Place a rolled blanket or a bolster lengthwise under your spine and have another prop, of lesser height, for your head. Settle on the blanket or bolster, bring your arms alongside the body, legs straight or knees up if that feels better for your back. Inhale, let your head slowly and gently drop back so that the crown of the head lands on the lower prop, feel that your throat and chest are wide open. If your neck is uncomfortable, the prop for the head needs to be higher. Breathe deeply. Stay as long as you wish, at least six long breaths if possible. To come out of the posture, either roll off the prop sideways, or tuck your chin in and press your hands on the floor on both sides of your body to sit up.

5

Neck stretch (*in pregnancy: from week 30 you can do this seated*).
Lying flat on the floor or with legs bent and knees up, cross your hands behind your head and bend your elbows. The whole weight of the head rests in the hands, the neck is relaxed. As you exhale lift your head and the top part of your shoulders (not the chest!) and take several deep breaths; you can turn your head to one side, then the other. End by softly resting the head back on the floor when your neck feels stretched enough.

6

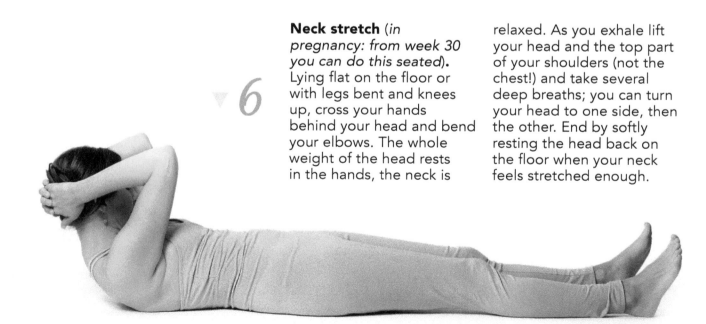

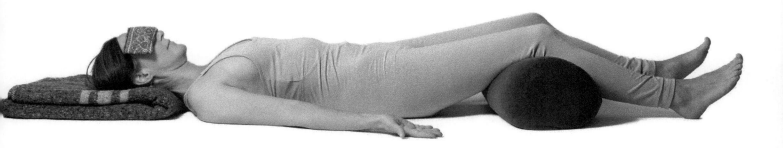

7

Rest: *Shavasana*, yoga's traditional resting pose (*in pregnancy, if over 30 weeks: lie on your side - common advice is the left side - with pillows under your head, between your knees and between your ankles*). Lying on the floor, make sure you are comfortable enough by having something slightly padded underneath you, at least a yoga mat or a blanket, especially looking after the area from the kidneys to the buttocks. Cover yourself with a blanket or a scarf, since the body cools down when it relaxes. If applicable, undo your belt and bra to be at ease. Place a flat pillow or folded scarf under your head to relax your neck. If the curve in your lower back is uncomfortable, place a pillow or rolled blanket under your knees. If your room is very bright, cover your eyes too.

Arms alongside the body, palms facing up, feet apart, relax your fingers and hands, toes and feet. To relax more deeply, practise three rounds of bumblebee breath (brahmari): mouth closed, inhale then exhale slowly, creating a humming sound in your throat like a "mmmm". Feel the vibration in your head, and rest in silence for at least 5 minutes.

MEDITATION
Resting in the light

Having found a comfy *shavasana* position, I imagine lying on warm sand, or in the fragrant grass of a summer meadow... All is well, I am in a calm atmosphere, this place suits me, I am at ease. I can feel all the parts of my body which are touching the floor: heels... calves... back of the thighs... buttocks... back... back of the shoulders... back of the head... touching the floor. I feel held and supported by Mother Earth. My muscles relax, since they have nothing to do. My breath is natural, free, easy. A ray of sunlight softly kisses my forehead. This ray of light seems to fill my head. With every inhalation a little more light enters my body. With every exhalation it seems to spread more inside of me. . Inhale, the light enters my head, exhale, the light fills my throat, and then my chest... another breath, light in my chest... as I keep breathing, it spreads down my arms, to the tips of my fingers. The light fills my belly, a lovely warm sensation, my belly is relaxed. Light spreads in my pelvis, my vagina... it travels down my legs, to the tips of my toes. My whole body is luminous, filled with light. I can feel that it is well, it is recharging. A bubble of light surrounds and protects me. I can stay here as long as I like.

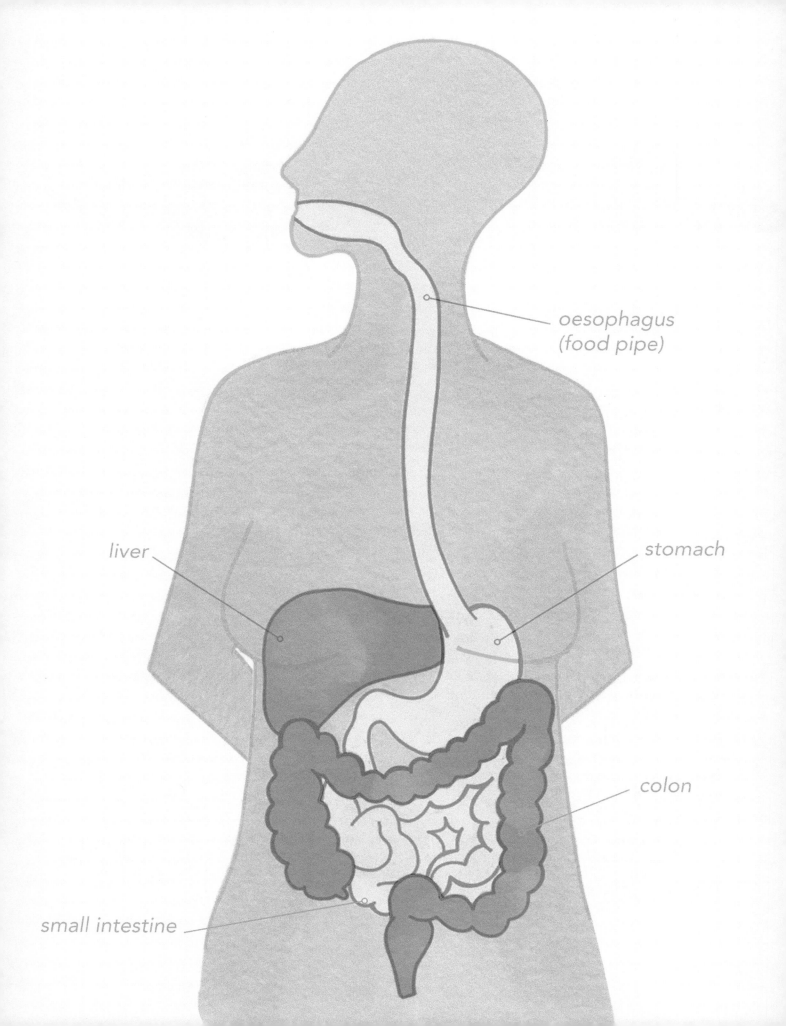

oesophagus
(food pipe)

liver

stomach

colon

small intestine

"The second brain": digestion, absorption, elimination

Every time you swallow something – a drink, a meal, or your lipstick – your digestion gets to work and selects: it takes what it needs straight away, stocks what it may need later, and eliminates the rest. Nutrients will be used to produce energy, and to grow or repair cells in order to survive. This is the basic digestive process when all goes well. However, when digestion is disrupted, the body will let you know: bloating, acid reflux, constipation… not to forget cellulite, acne, allergies, fertility issues, and even loss of bone density (osteoporosis).

The digestive system produces its own **gastro-intestinal hormones** (e.g. ghrelin, the "hunger hormone", and leptin, which manages appetite).
Furthermore, **the gut has its own nervous system, called "enteric" , aka the famous "second brain"**, which explains why your digestion is so important for emotions such as joy, anxiety, or even depression. This is due to neurotransmitters, particularly dopamine, which makes us chirpy in the mornings, and serotonin, which makes us feel happy and relaxed.

What's "normal" digestion?

It all begins in the **mouth**, before you even taste anything, because we salivate just by seeing or smelling a food item we like (even to think about it is enough!). Teeth and tongue will mince any food you take in your mouth and coat it with enzymes in your saliva, secreted by your salivary glands. **Hence why proper chewing is important.**
The food, prepared in this way, is swallowed and goes down to the stomach via the food pipe, aka the **oesophagus**.

In the **stomach**, hydrochloric acid and enzymes treat the food. The resulting mix then passes a sphincter, the pylorus, which is very sensitive to stress, to nervousness and to stimulants. A blockage of this sphincter causes vomiting. The food that was pre-treated by the stomach then enters the bowels. First it enters the **small intestine**, a narrow and very long tube (about 7 metres), before transiting into the **large intestine or colon**, which is wider but shorter (about 1,5 metres).

In the bowels, the food encounters bile and other digestive juices coming from the **gallbladder, the pancreas and the liver**, as well as the first part of our **gut flora, also called intestinal microbiota**, which encompasses a whole universe of bacteria, viruses, parasites and fungi.
Indeed, no matter how much you love your hygiene, our body is both covered and filled with bacteria. As professor Bernard David of the French Institute Pasteur writes, "from birth onwards, we live in a symbiosis with hundreds of billions of bacteria. [...] We find these micro-organisms everywhere in our body, even deep in our organs [...] (gut, skin, nose, ears, vagina, lungs, etc.)."[vi] All these organisms together form our **microbiome, which is as unique to each individual as their fingerprints.**

UNSUNG HEROES: 2

The vagus nerve

This long nervous pathway connects our brain with our gut, which is one of the reasons we call the digestive system the "second brain".

The vagus nerve originates in the head, travels down the neck and emerges at the front of the body at the level of the diaphragm. Its branches also reach the eyes and the glands in the brain, the mouth, the heart, the lungs, the whole digestive and urinary systems, the ovaries and the uterus.

The vagus nerve is involved in fainting episodes (sometimes with uncontrolled trembling) called "vasovagal episodes" which happen when the vagus nerves excessively lowers the blood pressure and slows the heartbeat too much.

Clinical trials proved that **stimulation of the vagus nerve creates an anti-inflammatory response** which could be used in treating chronic inflammation-based conditions such as Crohn's or rheumatoid arthritis . Stimulating the vagus nerve (by an electric implant) is already used to treat epilepsy and depression. **This will interest those wishing to regulate their body weight**: when the gut is full of food, especially

The inner wall of the gut absorbs the proteins and sugars which it transfers to the **liver** via the blood, and the liver transforms them again.

The liver purifies the blood and separates the nutrients from waste matter, which the bile then takes away if they can't be filtered through the kidneys. The larger molecules enter the **lymphatic system**, which is the "cleaning unit", and meets the venous circulation later. The "treatment centres" are the **lymph nodes**, of which many are found around the throat, in the armpits, and in the lower abdomen; they produce **antibodies, for our immunity**.

The kidneys allow the body to keep the steady level of hydration it needs. They filter your body's entire blood supply over the course of a day.

They also balance your mineral levels and **your acidity level**. If your food was too acidic, the excess will be eliminated to keep your blood at its ideal level, known as a "neutral blood pH".

The kidneys remove any substances from the blood that are potentially toxic and discard them into the urine, ending up in the **bladder before being eliminated via the urethra**, a pipe that exits the body through the pelvic floor.

In the colon, the waste matter that doesn't go through the kidneys is turned into the stool, which then goes into the end part of the colon, the rectum, where it will stay until expelled via the anus (also in the pelvic floor).

This entire digestive process from the mouth to the rectum takes between 8 hours and 3 days depending on the person, the type of food, and the circumstances.

As we had already seen in the part about the HPA axis, digestion is interrupted in case of stress, because the body focuses on providing energy to the arms and leg muscles to face danger (fight or flight). How can you repair the communication between the "two brains"? Now is the time to introduce you to the vagus nerve.

fats and proteins, the lining of the duodenum (the top part of the small intestine) produces cholecystokinin (CCK), a gut hormone, which has been studied for its capacity to regulate appetite and induce a feeling of being "full". It also raises the pain threshold. As it happens the vagus nerve is the one sending the message to the brain, which in return will produce oxytocin, the wellbeing hormone, which regulates trust and social behaviour. As you may have noticed in your daily life, **a full belly makes us feel calmer, more confident and more sociable**! This is exactly the rationale behind business lunches and family meals (it doesn't always work…).

It also explains why we tend to resort to food when we feel isolated or unsettled. Our body is just looking for a way to get its oxytocin "fix" in order to feel better. **A lack of pleasant social interactions, especially through touch, hugs or massages, therefore risks being compensated for via too much food intake, which the body will strain to digest**, creating imbalances. **Once you know this, check if you can give your body its oxytocin in a different way**, by interacting with friendly humans or pets.

The vagus nerve's transmission role can also be impeded by the position of your back (slouching too much), too much time spent on a chair rather than in a squatting position, or inflamed back muscles. This will impact digestion, hormone secretion, and even our state of mind (anxiety and depression). Any major deviations of the spine, such as scoliosis, a protruding neck ("text neck") and an excessive lumbar lordosis will also affect the vagus nerve.

Lastly, its pathway through the chest means it is affected by shallow breathing. **Breathing deeply and slowly stimulates the vagus nerve** (see the earlier breathing tip).

Other surprising ways to stimulate the vagus nerve:

○ Humming, like the bumblebee breath we saw in the first relaxation: when you hum, the vagus nerve connects with the vocal cords and is mechanically stimulated.
○ Splashing cold water on your face.
○ A big loud laugh (this is the whole idea of the method called "laughter yoga").

Women often suffer from various digestive issues, for hormonal reasons. Here are some classic ones you may well be familiar with:

The oesophageal sphincter, at the top of the stomach: if it is malfunctioning, you will suffer from **acid reflux**.

Certain hormones relax this sphincter, whose role it is to keep food from moving back up into the food pipe. This is often felt in pregnancy and therefore also tends to happen on the contraceptive pill. The pressure of the baby on the stomach can increase this opening of the sphincter in the "wrong" direction which causes the reflux. It has been measured that oestrogen and progesterone, given in perimenopause to decrease symptoms or improve bone density, also tend to cause reflux.[viii]

Acidic foods (meat and sugar) and lying flat tend to increase the reflux, it is therefore helpful to choose **alkaline foods** (vegetables, and some fruits) and to rest in a seated position after meals. Some women find that adding a tablespoon of apple cider vinegar (preferably organic and unpasteurised), or a teaspoon of bicarbonate of soda to a glass of room-temperature water and drinking it before bed, or first thing in the morning, helps.

Stomach: this is going to be a potential obstacle for those who have low levels of hydrochloric acid. This can have many causes: hypothyroidism, zinc deficiency, excessively sweet foods, eating on the go... your health care team may suggest taking digestive enzymes and hydrochloric acid as a supplement. Good results are also obtained again, with apple cider vinegar or lemon juice (diluted in water) or ginger (for example grated fresh into a hot drink).

Gut: the fluctuation of sexual hormones – testosterone and oestrogen – influence the content of the microbiota, which explains why digestion changes over the course of the menstrual cycle and digestive issues are common in perimenopause. Several studies have shown that certain bacteria of the gut flora improve anxiety **symptoms and depression**.[ix] Changes in the microbiota cause variations in the serotonin levels which several antidepressants then aim to correct.

Serotonin is mainly produced in the gut. It influences the body's temperature regulation, or behaviour around food and sex, our sleep, our pain threshold anxiety and movement.

Thought patterns (positive or negative) and physical exercise have an impact on its natural secretion. Natural daylight or light therapy (with special lamps) stop the transformation of serotonin to melatonin (the neurotransmitter of sleep), to avoid feeling drowsy during the day.

The microbiota also plays an essential role in inflammation, which in turn influences immunity: whilst a minimum of inflammation is necessary for the microbiota to function, big inflammatory reactions can be caused by an imbalance of this environment.

An immune reaction causes a localised inflammatory response and makes the gut lining more permeable; so certain substances reach the bloodstream where they can then create inflammation in other body parts such as the muscles, the liver, or the skin. This can create **inflammation-related conditions** such as Crohn's disease, but also diabetes and obesity, and even some tumours. Inflammation is also a suspected trigger for degenerative conditions such as Alzheimer's and Parkinson's.[x]

Irritable bowel syndrome (IBS) can appear in case of chronic inflammation of an imbalance in the gut flora or food intolerances. This can cause constipation, or its opposite, diarrhoea, which happens when the colon has not reabsorbed the liquid part of the food waste.

To look after your microbiota, make sure to eat a variety of good quality foods. That being said, the food's nutrients won't reach your cells if your body is unable to absorb them, and you may then eat the most local and organic foods without great effect. It is worth checking for food intolerances, parasites, or imbalances of the microbiota which are often caused by taking a course of antibiotics. A nutritionist or functional medicine practitioner can help you recover a healthy gut flora if you don't know how to do it.

Pancreas: it is both an organ of the digestive process and an endocrine gland. In its endocrine function, it synthetises hormones, in particular insulin (which lowers the blood sugar level) and glucagon (which raises it). Both influence the storage of glucose in the liver and therefore keep your blood sugar levels stable. An imbalance between those two hormones will eventually cause diabetes. There is proven link between thyroid disorders and blood sugar, showing that the thyroid has a role to play in this mechanism. This proves once more that the body should be considered as a whole and that it is worth checking the state of the digestive system in cases where hypo- or hyperthyroidism are diagnosed.

Oestrogen also influences blood sugar levels by affecting the cells of the pancreas and of the gut. This explains why type 2 diabetes is so frequent in women after menopause, whose oestrogen levels are lower, and why symptoms tend to improve when taking HRT (hormone replacement therapy).

Liver: an overburdened liver having to cope with food that is excessively fat, sweet, or artificial, as well as excessive alcohol consumption, often causes hormonal disruption, especially "oestrogen dominance" (too much oestrogen compared to the progesterone levels). The liver both produces and helps to transport several hormones or pre-hormones, which the adrenals, ovaries and thyroid then transform into hormones.
The liver has to work extra hard during the hormonal transition phases of puberty, pregnancy and perimenopause. The skin, in its function as an organ of elimination, will then tend to help evacuate the waste matters as pimples, which often indicate digestive issues.

Avoiding alcohol and choosing high-quality oils for cooking and seasoning both help the liver. It also benefits from dark green, bitter leaves (such as rocket), and freshly squeezed lemon juice diluted in warm water. **Herbalists offer good remedies to support the liver**, including artichoke, dandelion and milk thistle teas. They can advise you about right dosages and how to avoid interactions with any medication or other remedies you may be taking.

Kidneys: apart from acting as a filter, the kidneys also produce several hormones, enzymes and vitamins, such as Calcitriol, the active form of vitamin D, which allows the absorption of calcium by the gut and its storage in the bones. Healthy kidneys and a good level of vitamin D are therefore as important to prevent osteoporosis as calcium levels

are. Drinking sufficient quantities of water (as clean as possible) helps to prevent kidney stones and / or urinary tract infections. If you fail to drink enough, you will notice that the colour of your urine is a dark yellow, rather than a light straw colour.
If the kidneys are unable to keep the blood's acidity level in balance, the body may become "too acidic", which is called **metabolic acidosis**. The blood's pH may then still be "within the norm", but on the low side. As we age, the kidneys may struggle to keep that balance. Chronic acidosis can take hold. **Some doctors and nutritionists indeed consider "aging" to be, in effect, an acidification process, which then results in inflammation.**[xi]
Possible symptoms of acidosis are: strong body odour, fungal infections, kidney stones and urinary tract infections, high blood pressure, arteriosclerosis, demineralisation and osteoporosis, insulin resistance, tiredness and weight gain. Doctors don't always agree on the consequences of acidosis– except for osteoporosis. It has been proven that the body uses calcium stored in the bones to correct excess acidity. It is helpful to strive for a balance between acidic and alkaline foods if you have a family history of bone density issues.

Anus: If you often suffer from painful or uncomfortable excretion (chronic constipation), you may develop haemorrhoids, the anus may bleed, and the pelvic floor may lose its tone. It is useful to make sure that your stool is regularly expelled and comes out neither too hard, nor too watery.

How can you support your digestion?

Apart from the advice given in the section above, people who spend a lot of time seated certainly benefit from moving more, to activate motility, meaning bowel movements. Walking, taking the staircase, dancing, jumping with a rope, practicing yoga or Tai Chi… they all have the added advantage of reducing stress. On the other hand, people who regularly practise very demanding sports are actually in danger of adding more stress to their body. As we have seen, stress hinders the digestive process. So a good balance of movement and rest is what's needed to really benefit digestion.

KEEP YOUR BELLY WARM FOR OVERALL WELLBEING

by Tiffany Bown

Discover the benefits of a *Haramaki* and a belly blanket.

As soon as the weather gets colder, I'm taking more and more care to keep warm in my core. I know that staying warm here is the secret not only to feeling toasty all over, but also to feeling comfortable, supported, energised, creative and strong.

One of my favourite ways (on top of my Yoga and Qigong practice) of achieving this overall sense of well-being is wrapping my belly up with one of my much-loved 'Haramaki' cotton tubes or fleecy Cherishing Womb Wraps. If I'm feeling particularly in need of being held and nourished, I sometimes wear both.

Haramaki
Haramakis (translating literally as 'belly wrap') have been used for centuries in Japan. The word originally referred to a type of metal armour worn by soldiers in feudal Japan. More recently, these soft, stretchy tubes have been elevated to a fashion item in Japan, featuring bold designs to be worn on top of clothes. But simpler cotton versions are still worn under clothes for their health benefits, covering from the Kidneys to lower back or hips. Several different brands are now available in Europe – including original Japanese ones (I have a Kokoro Haramaki) and Western variations (I have a Tube by Harry Duley).

Cherishing Belly Blanket
These are long pieces of fabric designed to be worn over clothes, wrapping and tying around your middle. They are made in a range of colours in cosy fleece (for the Winter) or pretty cotton (for the summer). The Winter ones even

have a little pocket in the back to hold a hot water bottle (which can feel so soothing during Moontime). These lovely wraps are made by Claire Taylor at Cherishing Everything.

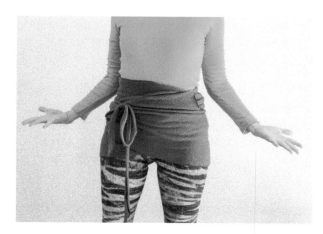

Why keep your midriff warm?
Because it keeps you warm and there are numerous health benefits, but also because it just feels so deliciously good and right to be held here. Even better than you might imagine or than I can describe – perhaps because us women are always running around supporting others, so our bodies take a big grateful sigh at this supportive gesture of self-care.
The only way to find out how a Haramaki feels is to try one.

Key for our health, fertility and creative power
Here's a closer look at why keeping our midriffs warm with wraps is so important for our health and well-being – and why exposing our tender centre to the cold (as is the scary fashion trend among teenage girls) does us such great harm. Haramakis and other belly wraps cover:

○ **our Kidneys**, which are the guardians of the original energy we received when we were conceived, thus the source of the energy that animates all other organs and tissues. They are like the batteries of our body. Cold drains their energy, thereby depleting our overall reserves. When our Kidneys get cold, it is like the fire going out in our system, so we always feel cold and lose our motivating drive. Worse still, as the Kidneys are the organs most intimately connected to our female sexual health, Coldness leads to all kinds of reproductive system problems, including low libido and fertility issues.

○ **our vital energy centre** (*Hara* in Japanese or Lower *Dantian* in Chinese), located two inches below the navel and back into the centre of the abdomen. The Lower *Dantian* provides the driving force to circulate energy around our body. Coldness here is a sign of low vital energy and causes stagnation in our core, so whatever energy we do have does not circulate freely. This, in turn, affects our blood circulation. As a result, we feel cold, weak, tired, apathetic and slide into ill-health.

○ **our womb** – our Womb space is closely linked to our Kidney energy. A 'Cold Womb' is one of the key patterns underlying infertility in Chinese medicine. But our Womb is not only a cradle for physical babies; it is the source of all our creative and nurturing power as women. When we allow this sacred space within us to freeze over, we lose our capacity to connect with this gentle, yet unstoppable, strength in our centre. In addition, Cold stagnation in our Womb is a cause of painful menstrual cramps.

○ **our lower back** – pain in the lower back is often a sign of Kidney energy imbalance.

○ **our small and large intestines** - internal Cold makes it very hard for our digestive system to do its job of digesting food. It results in sluggishness, leading to pain, constipation, loose stools and other symptoms of digestive disharmony.

So the health of our whole body depends on being warm in our centre.

But these wraps cannot do miracles. If we continue with other habits that let the cold in, our body will continue to struggle to maintain its warmth – and to heal or fend off the imbalances mentioned above.

Other tips to nurture your internal warmth

○ **If you get cold, get warm** – this may seem obvious, but it's important to know that when you are cold, your energy is contracting and stagnating further, further heightening your greater tendency to feel cold (and lethargic etc).

○ **Keep your feet, hands and head warm** – in addition to your middle, it is also particularly easy to be attacked by the Cold through your hands, feet and head, so take care to keep them warm. Be sure to avoid walking on cold floors, else a key energy point on your soles will take that coldness straight to your centre and your Womb space. And try not to sit or lie on those cold floors either. I also highly recommend keeping your wrists and calves warm, as you'll feel chilled all over if you get cold here.

○ **Don't swim during your Moontime** – the Chinese never swim when menstruating because the Womb (ie the cervix) is 'open', so it is particularly susceptible to being invaded by the Cold.

○ **Avoid cold food and drinks and raw food** – one of the key ways that we chill our system is by consuming food and drink straight from the fridge. This compromises the hot stomach's capacity to start the digestive process, and an energy point in the mouth takes the Cold straight to the *Dantian* energy centre in our abdomen. Raw food has a cooling and weakening effect on the body. So food is generally best eaten at least lightly cooked – and, when the weather is cold, long-cooked hearty soups and stews are wonderful for nourishing and keeping warm. Ice-cream is one of the worst things you could possibly eat – combining cold, sugar and fat. Sorry!

Take a few minutes to relax whilst soaking up magnesium to help with fatigue, anxiety, period pain, perimenopause symptoms, calf muscle cramps, insomnia, or osteoporosis.

The skin is both a natural barrier and an organ which can both excrete and absorb. Soaking up nutrients through your skin is the principle behind all "skin patches" (such as the ones to help kick a smoking habit or administer small doses of oestradiol). Studies on these transdermal patches show that heating the skin increases absorption of the active substances.[xii]

So let's **raise our magnesium intake. Stress, sugar and coffee contribute to lowering magnesium levels in the bloodstream, and poor soil quality also means our food doesn't contain much of it. Yet this mineral is crucial for women's health**, and with our hectic Western lifestyle, most of us don't get enough of it. It helps against muscle cramps, fosters relaxation, strengthens bones, and is needed by the thyroid, as well as regulating blood sugar, iron absorption and the production of sexual hormones.

It's easy: **fill a foot basin or bucket with warm/ hot water and add about a cup of magnesium flakes** (magnesium chloride - I like the quality label "Zechstein Inside") which will dissolve in the water. Epsom salts (magnesium sulphate), can be a cheaper alternative. You may want to add a few drops of calming essential oils, such as lavender or frankincense. **Sit comfortably on a chair or sofa and soak your feet for approximately 20 minutes**.

This foot bath is ok for pregnant women, with a lower dosage of flakes you'll find on the packaging (but pregnant women should avoid essential oils).

Obviously, your body will absorb the magnesium even if you read or watch TV while you sit there. Yet if you want to make the most of this time, you could practise deep breathing, listen to calming music or an inspiring podcast, massage some nice cream or oil into your face, or meditate. That way you can turn these 20 minutes into a real wellness break. After drying your feet, take the opportunity to moisturise them, massaging any tender areas. Then slip on some cotton or woollen socks, and if you can go to bed straight away, you may well enjoy a good night's sleep!

A MASSAGE
For a healthy belly

This massage supports digestion and can help with premenstrual syndrome and period pain. You can choose any natural oil you like (without endocrine disruptors!). Ayurveda recommends castor oil for its anti-inflammatory virtues. This colourless oil is also used to nourish hair, nails and eyelashes. Dr Christiane Northrup recommends it for womb poultice to help with menstrual cramps. It is rather sticky, a bit less so when heated. Sweet almond oil is another common base oil for massages.

Several scientific studies have proven that oil massages with a few drops of lavender and clary sage essential oil added to the base, do help with cramping . Whilst these studies have used different dosages, just bear in mind that a few drops should be enough. Make sure you are not allergic to these oils by testing them beforehand on your wrist or inner elbow.

This massage can be done seated or lying down, just protect any surfaces or bedlinen with a towel.

1) Pour about one finger of your base oil and a few drops of essential oils in a glass, and stand the glass in a bowl with hot water to gently heat the oil.

2) Dip your fingers into the warm oil and rub your hands to distribute it evenly. You can always dip your fingers back in throughout the massage to add some more. Place both hands flat on your belly, under your ribcage, on your right side where your liver is, leave them there a moment, then massage the whole belly by rotating in the same direction as your digestion: from the liver, cross over to the left side under your ribs, then down above your left hip then cross again to the lower right side, and come back up to the liver, and repeat approximately 20 times.

3) Then change technique, still rotating in the same direction, but this time grabbing a bit of skin and belly fat with your fingers as if kneading dough with your hands.

4) Now place your hands flat on the lower part of your belly, fingers pointing down, and rub up and down on your hip creases, your groin.

5) To conclude, rest with your hands flat on your belly, feeling their warmth, breathing deeply.

Yoga sequence for digestion

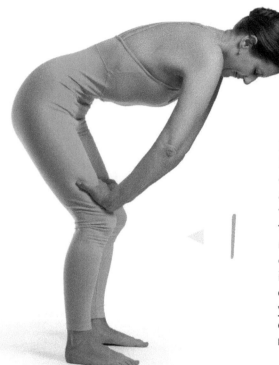

◀ 1

X! Abdominal lock.
Standing or seated, inhale deeply through the nose and then bend down vigorously whilst exhaling, to empty your lungs as much as possible. On empty lungs, so without inhaling again, lift your chest half way and press your hands into your thighs, elbows bent. Tuck your navel in and lift it, as if to tuck it under your ribcage, there is a sensation of air having been sucked out, this can sometimes also be felt in the throat. When you feel the need to inhale, lift your chest and inhale slowly, relaxing the belly. Just do it once if you are new to this, otherwise practise three in a row, preferably in the morning, since it is energising!

▶ 2

Squat (*OK in prenatal except if the placenta is under the baby. Avoid in the postnatal phase*).
If your knees are sensitive, sit on a bolster or big cushion. Enter this pose from a standing position by bending your knees and bringing your hips down as far as they can go, legs apart. Your feet can point outwards if this feels better for you. Sit in your squat with elbows bent, arms pressing against the insides of your legs, and hands in prayer for the more active version. In the more relaxed version, let your arms come down to the floor, between your legs. If your heels don't touch the floor, roll up a blanket and place it under them. Stay as long as you can. To leave the posture, just bring your buttocks to the floor and extend your legs in front of you.

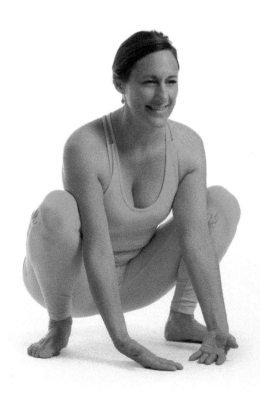

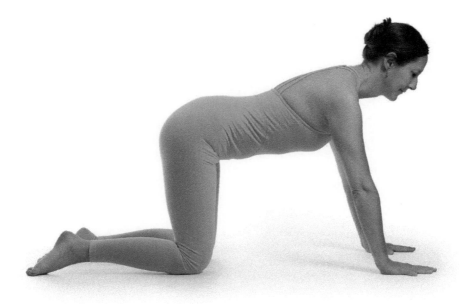

3 All fours.
Come unto all fours, hands under your shoulders, or slightly in front of them if you have long arms and a long upper body compared to your legs. Knees hip-width apart, toes pointing back, keep your lower back flat (avoid a deep downward tilt of the lumbar spine). Place a blanket under your knees for added comfort.

4 X! The tiger and the balancing table.
From the all fours position, extend your right leg behind you, toes on the floor, heel stretching back. Raise your left arm and hold it parallel to the floor, at shoulder height. Engage your abdominal muscles to feel stable. Now, on an inhalation, lift the back leg by activating your thigh and gluteus muscles; bring the leg parallel to the floor or a bit higher. As you exhale, tuck your navel in, bend your right knee and bring it forward, as you bow the head down and bring the left elbow in to meet the right knee, rounding the back. Inhale returning to the previous extended position. Repeat three times if this is new for you, 6 to 10 times once you are used to it, then change sides and repeat the same number of times. Keep your shoulder muscles active by really pushing the floor away with the supporting hand and arm.

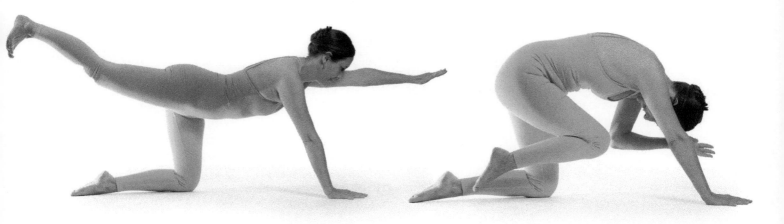

Child's pose
(prenatal: legs wide to make space for the baby). From all fours, stretch back to bring your buttocks towards your heels. If they don't quite reach, place a blanket or cushion between heels and buttocks. Bow your head down. If it doesn't touch the floor, make fists with your hands and rest the forehead on the fists.

Stay in this position and enjoy the stretch in the lower back. Breathe deeply, focusing on your back. To come out of the posture, slowly unfurl your back to sit up.

▼5

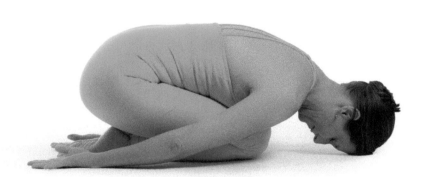

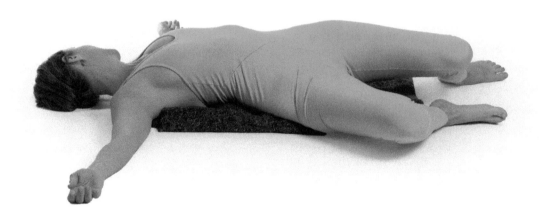

X! Supine twist.
▲6

Lie on your back, knees bent, feet on the floor. Place some padding under your head if needed, you may also want a blanket under your hips and lower back. Spread your arms wide, on the floor, at approximately shoulder height. There are several options for your feet:

they can be hip width apart or wider, on the edges of the mat, they can be close to the buttocks, or further down. Try several positions to find the one that suits you best. Inhale, then on the exhalation drop your knees to the right. Inhale as you bring the knees back up. Exhale as you drop them to the left, and keep

going in this way for as long as you like. If it's ok for your neck, you can turn your head in the opposite direction to your knees. After several repetitions of the active version of the posture, you can stay on one side, for 5 or 10 breaths, and then change sides and stay there for the same amount of time.

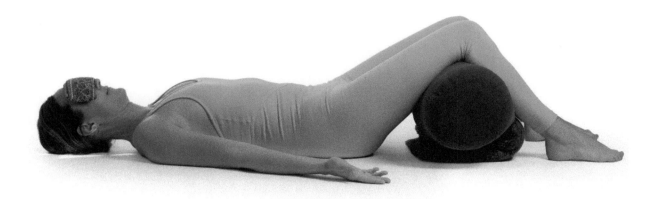

7

Rest: constructive rest pose, supported version. Lying on the floor, supporting your head and hips as needed, place bolsters or pillows under your knees to keep them up like a triangle whilst you relax completely (your feet are on the floor). The back is on the floor, with just a slight natural upward curve in the lower back. Breathe deeply, feeling your ribcage expand sideways and up as you inhale, and lowering down on the exhale. You could initially place your hands on your ribs to feel them moving – outwards on the inhalation, inwards on the exhalation. Then relax your arms alongside the body, palms facing up. Turn your head from side to side a couple of times then place your face up, and rest, with your eyes closed or open as you choose, and feel your breath like waves. Your back relaxes completely. Stay as long as you wish, and when you feel like leaving the posture, draw your knees towards your chest, place your hands on the bolster or pillows to push them away, and roll to your side. Support yourself with your hands pressing into the floor to slowly sit up again.

MEDITATION
Mindful food tasting

According to your preference, choose a raisin, an olive, a piece of chocolate… Sit in a comfortable position, in a calm space where you will not be disturbed. Take the food item you chose in your hand, have a good look at its colours, then close your eyes. Begin by feeling the item in your palm. Then bring it up to your nose to smell it. Now open your lips and place it in your mouth. Examine it with your tongue, rolling it against the roof of your mouth. Notice its taste and texture. Feel the saliva forming in your mouth. If any memories associated with this food come up, acknowledge them kindly without dwelling on them, since what you want is to focus on this moment right now. Try to keep the morsel of food in your mouth as long as possible. If it is one that doesn't melt, you'll end up chewing it. Observe again. Then swallow it, feel it travel down your food pipe and imagine it arriving in your stomach, which has prepared the right juices to start digesting it. Later, your body will break down the nutrients and carry them to your cells to nourish them, and the waste will be eliminated. Everything you swallow has an effect on your body, your mood, your energy level, your overall health. Take as much time as you like to contemplate this.

"Womanhood": womb, ovaries, vagina, and breasts

Most women have little choice: their family and/or their employer expect the same level of engagement from them, day in, day out. Yet the female body experiences considerable hormonal fluctuations over the course of the menstrual cycle which have a strong effect on mood and energy levels. Our health pays the price of a standardised lifestyle which would be better suited to a machine than to a real human being!

These cyclical variations, especially menstrual bleeding, are often considered a "nuisance" or even a "curse", and yet menstrual bleeding is beneficial: **by shedding the endometrium, the uterus, in a way, "self-cleans". Every month, it regenerates itself and starts anew**.

Obviously, those of you who suffer from premenstrual syndrome (PMS), heavy cramps, or are trying to conceive a baby, may not be entirely at peace with your cycle. Taking anti-inflammatories every month is not a sustainable solution for cramps, since they are not without side-effects.

Your food, the quality of your rest, an adequate amount of movement and all the other things that happen in your life over the course of a month, will influence the days before and during your period: sometimes the experience can be rather sweet, with a regular flow and hardly any pain. Sometimes PMS symptoms will show up as anger or frustration, the first day of bleeding may be really painful and the flow dark, thick, or exhaustingly abundant. **Every month, you get a chance to make choices that will help your body be more balanced**.

The persisting taboos around menstruation aren't helpful in confronting problems head on to find solutions and heal. **Yet a great many women are able to improve the way they experience menstruation, pregnancy, and perimenopause by combining stress relief, suitable movement and adequate nutrition**. Even if this seems obvious to you, I can assure you that it is still news to many women who come to consult myself and the other specialists in this book. Always remember, you are not condemned to suffering, and it certainly is not "God's will".

It is wonderful to be a woman. We all deserve to flourish in our femininity and to reconnect with this "nest" we have in us, the womb, the seat of our creativity.

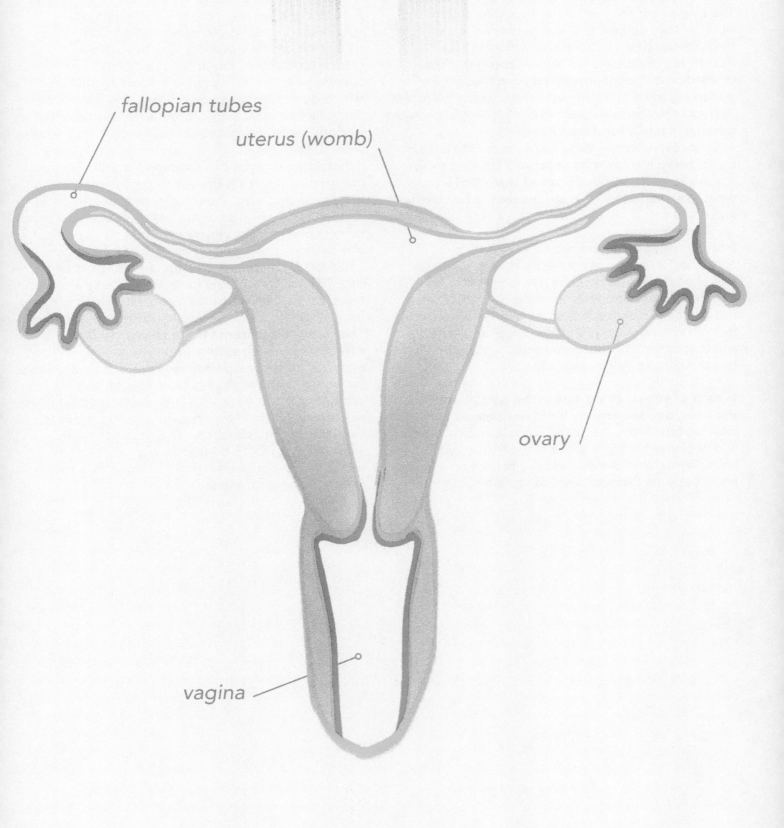

fallopian tubes

uterus (womb)

ovary

vagina

The ovaries are gonads (sexual glands), they produce oocytes (eggs) which could become babies. The ovaries are also part of the endocrine system, because they synthesise sexual hormones, in particular oestrogen and progesterone, as well as smaller quantities of testosterone. We saw above that the production of these hormones is controlled by the pituitary gland and the hypothalamus via the hormones FSH and LH. Messages are constantly being exchanged between the head and the lower belly.

At birth, every female baby has a stock of follicles, this is called the "**ovarian reserve**". Until recently, it was also **generally understood that all of a woman's ovarian follicles are present at her birth** and could only diminish in number with age, all the way up to menopause.

Scientific research conducted in 2004-2005 by Jonathan Tilly's team question this dogma. They say that adult ovaries do produce new oocytes.[xiv] This notion of "**neo-oogenesis**" is still subject to debate, but I chose to mention it to show you that we are still far from knowing everything about women's fertility, and that those "conception miracles" you may have heard about are indeed possible.

In case of stress, as we saw in the part about the axes, ovarian activity is either "paused" or interrupted, which affects the entire hormonal balance, and of course fertility. It is one of the reasons your libido (sexual desire) may suddenly flourish on holidays, and a baby may appear nine months after your trip!

Polycystic ovaries syndrome, or PCOS, is the most frequent hormonal issue for women of fertile age. A blood analysis will reveal it, as will an ultra-sound scan. Indeed, its name comes from one of this syndrome's aspects which is visible on ultra-sound scans: multiple little "cysts" around the ovaries. These "cysts" are actually follicles which don't begin to grow during the last part of the follicular phase. PCOS will lead to irregular periods, acne, excess facial hair and, in its extreme form, infertility.

Whilst the origin of this condition is still controversial it is clearly associated with hyperandrogenism, meaning excess secretion of "male" hormones, and insulin resistance. Doctors usually prescribe hormones to treat it, in particular the contraceptive pill, or, in case of infertility, CLOMID (clomiphene citrate), an anti-oestrogen drug. These treatments have side-effects and don't treat the root cause of the problem, which is the hormonal imbalance requiring lasting re-balancing. **"Natural" treatments have shown to be effective by addressing lifestyle issues**, especially via stress reduction, correcting digestive problems, and stabilising blood sugar levels. Women such as Alisa Vitti (see. bibliography) have written about their own natural healing process, over-riding their doctor's initial scepticism. By addressing a PCOS diagnosis in your younger fertile years, you are setting sail towards a more serene perimenopause.

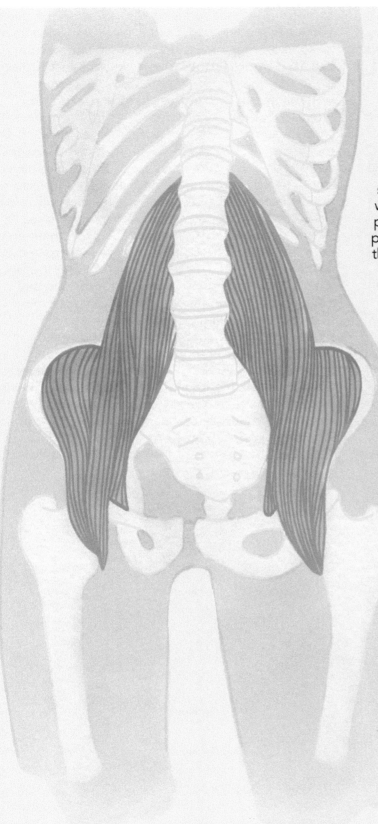

UNSUNG HEROES: 3

The psoas

What we call "the psoas", is actually two pairs of muscles: the psoas major, which connects the spine with the inner thighs, and the psoas minor, which connects the spine to the pelvis (some people don't have a psoas minor). Both sets of psoas muscles create a group on each side of the pelvis, together with the iliacus muscle, which connects the pelvis and the legs. These are crucial muscles for posture, since they connect the upper and the lower body, allowing us to walk.

The psoas connects with the diaphragm at the level of the T12 vertebra, an area also known as the **solar plexus**.

Since the psoas runs through the belly and pelvis, it influences digestion and the sexual organs. When it is not in good shape, this can manifest as backache, period pain, or constipation. Physical inactivity (spending your days seated on chairs, sofas etc., rather than alternating between squats, sitting on your heels, and sitting cross-legged) affects the psoas by "shortening" and stiffening it. Pregnancy can also be a stressor for the psoas, as well as the scar tissue of a caesarean section. Osteopathy and myofascial release therapy can help with the psoas.

Constructive rest pose, lying on your back with your knees bent and feet flat on the floor, brings relief to the psoas. You can enhance it with small pelvic tilts (flatten the lower back into the floor on the exhalation and gently arch it on the inhalation), by bridge pose, by coming onto all fours, the balancing on one knee and one hand, and by practising backbends such as the sphinx, as well as shavasana. You will find these poses in the yoga sequence.

There is quite a bit of confusion around this topic, so let's check a few facts. Menopause is the end of the reproductive phase in a woman's life, generally happening around the age of 50 (this is an average – it can happen any time from your late thirties to your early sixties). The ovaries gradually stop producing sexual hormones (oestrogen and progesterone), ovulation no longer takes place, and there are no more periods.

When the ovaries diminish and eventually stop their oestrogen production, the adrenal glands and the fatty tissue will keep making small quantities of it. **This is why women tend to gain weight around the belly in their forties and fifties**, as we saw in the chapter about the HPO axis. A little bit of weight gain may therefore help you to enjoy the benefits of oestrogen for longer (better mood, bone density, skin elasticity and hydration), whereas too much weight gain will cause problems, due to excess oestrogen in proportion to progesterone.

Medically speaking, a woman has experienced menopause when she has gone without a period for 12 consecutive months.

The time before and after this date, when ovulation becomes erratic and oestrogen levels vary (sometimes like a roller-coaster) is perimenopause.

Symptoms will not suddenly disappear on the day you reach menopause. During those transition years, all sorts of more or less uncomfortable symptoms can appear: hot flushes, digestive issues, disrupted sleep patterns, mood swings, poor concentration, unstable joints, dryness, sagging skin, etc. The intensity of those symptoms varies from woman to woman: some will literally just stop menstruating and that's it, whilst others can have moderate to severe symptoms (20 to 30% of women). Those who have experienced motherhood may often be surprised to find sensations and issues reappear which will remind them of their pregnancy and post-partum days.

As we saw in the chapter about the axes, there are effective natural methods to help you navigate this hormonal transition, and if you are reading this book in your thirties, know that looking after yourself now will help prepare your body and your mind for this peculiar phase in a woman's life.

By the way, there is no reason to stop feeling like a 'real woman' (nor to stop being sexually active!) when you reach menopause. **For many women, their fifties mark the beginning of one of their freest and most creative phases**. With an average life expectancy of 81 years for women in the UK, you still have one third of your life ahead of you to benefit from all the experience accumulated by that time!

Here are two simple and useful tricks for when you feel submerged by a heatwave due to hormonal fluctuations (pregnancy and perimenopause in particular).

Shitali – the serpent breath
This traditional yoga practice, used to cool down when it gets too hot, works well for hot flushes.
Some of us can roll up the sides of their tongue to create a little tube, others can't (apparently it's genetic!). The traditional version prescribes making the tube, but to replace that, you can just softly place your tongue between your upper and lower rows of teeth.
So roll up your tongue or place it between your teeth, then inhale through the mouth as if through a straw. The air will feel fresh on your tongue.
Then close your mouth and exhale slowly through the nose.

If you are NOT pregnant, you can pause at the end of the inhalation and keep the air inside for a brief moment to enhance the effect.
Pregnant women should not hold their breath.
Repeat this breathing pattern at least three times – you will feel its effect immediately, but it does dry out the mouth a little, so don't overdo it, especially if you tend to have a dry mouth, or drink a few sips of water afterwards (at room temperature, not icy).

Ear stimulation
Simultaneously pinch the top of both ears between your thumb and index fingers of each hand, so right hand on right ear and vice-versa.
Go around both ears from top to bottom pinching in this way. Your pinch can be quite firm. Once you come near the lobes, turn your hands around so you can hold them firmly to pull them down. Pull the lobes downwards three times. Your ears will be red and feel hot, and yet funnily enough, this can help cool a hot flash.

Dry and tired eyes are due to screen-based work (not enough blinking when you stare at the screen so humidity evaporates), **contact lenses, smoking** (the smoke attacks the cornea) **and air conditioning. Dry eyes are a problem which particularly affects women in perimenopause, since hormonal changes can cause overall dryness.**

For a quick fix:

- **blink** to hydrate the eye (without contact lenses): open your eyes wide, then blink them shut and open them again quickly, about ten times. Then keep your eyes closed for a few breaths. Repeat for another two cycles.
- **Palming**: bring the palms of your hands together and rub them to create heat. Close your eyes, cup your hands and place them over your eyes without pushing against the eyeballs. Open your eyes to gaze into these dark, warm caves. Repeat as often as you like.

Additionally, when you are at home, Ayurveda recommends **massaging around the eyes** (on the bones, under the eyebrows, and on the temples) **with tiny circular movements**. Do this massage with your fingertips, which you will have dipped in warm sesame oil, and then gently remove it with a cotton pad dipped in (organic) rose water, which creates a pleasant fresh sensation. You could recline and rest for a few minutes with the rose water cotton pads over your eyes.

The womb

The uterus, or womb as it is commonly known in English, is an organ which looks like a pouch, and has many blood vessels running through it. It is open at the bottom, where you find the **cervix**. Towards the back, two separate parts branch out into the Fallopian tubes, which connect it to the ovaries. The uterus is lined with a membrane, the uterine endometrium, which changes according to the messages it receives via the ovarian hormones.

As we saw in the chapter on the axes, from puberty to menopause, a woman with relatively balanced hormones will menstruate about once a month. During the first part of the menstrual cycle, the lining keeps thickening, preparing to receive the ovum, the "egg". If the egg is not fertilised, the lining will be shed during menstruation.

Fertility

Wishing for a baby and not seeing that wish come true creates stress, sadness, even despair, and is one of the motivations (sometimes a necessity) which brings women to develop more interest in their body and rethink their lifestyle.

In the commented bibliography at the end of this book, you will find several titles, quite different from each other, which specifically address this topic and offer tried and tested approaches, such as Jani White's book, which emphasises the fertility of the couple and invites both partners to be involved.

Natural methods, and in particular acupuncture, tend to work really well in all those cases where a medical examination has not revealed any physical obstacles, such as blocked tubes.

I mentioned more than once already how stress and nutrition affect fertility. Your body and subconscious mind may block conception if they sense a situation of "chronic scarcity" – such as lack of sleep, of moral support, of safety, of vitamins… Rika Lukac, a yoga teacher and nutritionist who specialises in fertility (see bibliography), lists six physical stress factors:

- dehydration
- fluctuations of blood sugar levels
- too much acidity
- an overburdened liver

- an imbalance in the gut flora
- depleted levels of micro- and macronutrients.

Whilst this list mainly encourages you to review what you eat and drink, emotional stress also affects acidity, the liver and nutrient uptake. In the case of stress, the adrenals also use progesterone to create stress hormones, rather than favouring the implantation of the fertilised egg, as we saw in the chapter on the axes.

Even if you are just starting out on your fertility journey, remember that **traditional medical systems, and in particular Ayurveda, advise for both partners to start preparing consciously several months before they even begin to try conceiving**. Indeed, Ayurveda reminds us that spermatogenesis, the production of sperm which may fertilise the ovum, takes around two and a half months. To optimise their chances of conceiving a strong and healthy baby, both the man and woman can start by eliminating toxins from their body, then follow a healthy lifestyle for several months and "invite" the baby by consuming specific tonics, called vajikaranas, as well as freeing up space and time for this child to enter their lives.
Yoga, which offers movements to avoid stagnation in the pelvis and encourages relaxation, has also helped many women conceive.

Motherhood

The fact that another human being is created and grows within a woman's womb is both magical and fascinating. **As far as hormones are concerned, pregnancy and the postnatal phase cause a massive upheaval**, which explains the emotional roller-coaster these women can find themselves on, between bliss, tenderness, anxiety, and depression (both before and after birth). The "negative" emotions are often hard for both the mum and her community to accept, especially if the pregnancy was long-awaited. Yet the whole range of feelings is normal.
Progesterone is produced in great quantities all through pregnancy, first by the corpus luteum, then by the placenta. Oestrogen levels explode, providing the increase in blood volume needed to supply the baby with nutrients and oxygen. The sudden rise of hormone levels can cause nausea, especially in early pregnancy (a tablespoon of apple cider vinegar diluted in a glass of water may help). Constipation, a well-known issue for many pregnant women, is also hormone-related.

Moving often, but without excess, for example by joining a prenatal yoga class, helps to encourage bowel motility. It will also prevent back pain and prepare the body for giving birth.
Gestational diabetes, checked by a glucose tolerance test, can also be due to the hormonal fluctuations which influence the blood sugar levels (acupuncture has a good track record for this).
The womb widens to accommodate the growing foetus. Muscles and ligaments of the belly stretch. The hormone relaxin prepares the pelvis to help with baby's passage during birth, but makes other joints (like wrists, knees, and ankles) unstable at the same time. The back and legs must get used to carrying a heavier load. The breasts swell.
During labour, progesterone levels plummet, which enables contractions to begin. The cervix opens, the vagina dilates to make way for baby. Other hormones are involved in labour: oxytocin brings on contractions and numbs pain together with endorphins, and finally, an adrenalin peak will usher in the final phase. Contractions in the womb help expulse the baby. After both the baby and then the placenta are delivered, uterine muscles will retract (which will be facilitated by breastfeeding) and the womb will slowly return more or less to its pre-pregnancy size.

After giving birth, hormone levels will return to their pre-conception levels, except for prolactin and oxytocin, which allow breastfeeding and bonding with baby. The drop in hormone levels can be quite brutal and exhausting.
As we have seen throughout this book, hormones affect mood, and it is therefore normal for the young mother to fluctuate from laughing to crying in a minute, and she may even experience "baby blues", anxiety, anger or sometimes even severe depression. This is nothing to be ashamed of. It can be quite normal not to feel as happy as you think you should be, so make sure you surround yourself with a network of helpful and supportive people, and do seek professional help if things feel really bad. Remember to check your thyroid, which can become imbalanced during pregnancy because of the links between the three axes.
The elements of "rest" and "connection" are equally important, yet not always taken into account in our society. Many women need to (or think they should) "function like before" quite quickly after giving birth. One reason is that they often need to get back to work relatively soon, the other is that they would like to regain their pre-pregnancy physique. In Asian cultures women are expected to rest for several weeks after giving birth,

during which other women will help out with household tasks. Special nourishing dishes are prepared for the new mother, and she is assisted in tying a sarong or a scarf around her belly to compensate for this weird sensation of emptiness or heaviness which can appear after the baby has left the womb.

If you feel lonely, out of sorts, or overwhelmed, this is not surprising, and you may benefit from joining a group of other new mums, for postnatal yoga for instance, in order to feel the support of the group, to exchange information, and to enjoy some safe stretching and gentle toning. Neglecting the postnatal phase is good neither for you, nor for your baby, who needs a mum who is at peace in both her body and mind.

Avoid taking up normal abdominal toning exercises too quickly, especially anything that requires you to lift the chest and shoulders from a position where you are lying on your back. You want to prevent consolidating a separation of your rectus abdominis muscles (the ones which were stretched apart by your growing belly). On the other hand, lying on the floor for some stretches and twists, with deep exhales during which you bring the navel in towards the spine and lift it towards the ribs, will help to reknit your abdominal muscles.

In France, unlike the UK, perineal (and abdominal) rehabilitation after pregnancy is offered by the national health system. This is useful even after a caesarean section, because the baby will still have weighed on your pelvic floor and stretched your belly muscles during the pregnancy. You may also benefit from practicing the pelvic floor breath described in this book (see the chapter on the pelvic floor).

Birth control

Presenting the pros and cons of each and every contraceptive method would go beyond the scope of this book. I just want to remind you, especially the younger women, that you have various options, despite the fact that the situation is often presented to you like a binary choice between the pill and condoms.

In principle, there are two types of contraceptive products: those that affect the ovarian hormones, the HPO axis, by adding synthetic hormones into the bloodstream (the pill, the patch, implants, the IUD with added hormones…), and those which create a physical barrier (the male condom, the cap, the copper IUD), which do not interfere with the natural hormone cycle. Tubal ligation, whilst being a physical intervention and not a hormone addition, does have some influence on the ovaries' natural cycle.

Obviously, the one method that also protects from sexually transmitted diseases is the male condom.

A word on taking the pill "back to back", for several months without the week of interruption, so that periods do not occur: it is obviously up to you, after discussing it with your gynaecologist, whether this may be a good idea in your case. From the point of view of natural healing methods, periods are considered to be times when the womb "cleans itself" and a chance to take stock of how your lifestyle choices in the past month have impacted you. Let us not forget, however, that most women who have access to contraception will have many more periods over their lifetime than women did even just a hundred years ago, when they were generally either pregnant or lactating during most of their fertile years. We therefore bleed more often than they did, which may cause deficiencies (particularly in iron levels), which may need monitoring.

Your period pain may be caused by **endometriosis**. This is a condition whereby cells from the endometrium travel from the womb towards other body parts, via the Fallopian tubes. The tissue which then grows outside the womb causes lesions, adhesions, and cysts (endometrioma) in or around the affected organs.

Whilst the cause of endometriosis is still being researched, there does seem to be a genetic factor, since it often affects several generations of women within the same family.

An excessively high level of oestrogen is another one of the main theories being explored. The following factors can raise the oestrogen level above the average level:

∘ fewer pregnancies.

∘ being overweight – as we have seen, fatty tissue, especially around the belly, can create oestrogen.

∘ Eating red meat has been scientifically proven to be an aggravating factor, whereas fruit and vegetables seem to have a positive effect.[xv]

∘ Stress is considered by some experts to be an aggravating factor.[xvi]

Endometriosis currently affects *at least* 1 in 10 women and will cause different symptoms, with excruciating period pain, chronic fatigue, pain during intercourse and very heavy blood flow for some, whilst others are hardly aware of it. EndoFrance, the French endometriosis charity, reports that "nowadays, **endometriosis is often diagnosed by chance and with an average delay of five years**, during which the condition may have caused damage to the affected organs". It often remains undiagnosed until the woman goes for a fertility check-up, since it can have a negative impact on conception (infertility in 30 to 50 % of cases). If these symptoms sound familiar, you may want to insist on being tested for endometriosis, as a surprising number of GPs are still not very familiar with the condition.

The list above shows you that there are several factors which you can target simultaneously if you fine-tune your diet and address your stress.

In combination with traditional methods such as acupuncture, very good results are often obtained. If that should not prove to be enough, doctors nowadays tend to prescribe other treatments that can be quite severe but are sometimes necessary: taking the pill 'back to back' to avoid getting a period; provoking an artificial menopause by taking hormones which impact the HPO axis; and in some cases surgery, which can go from "cleaning" the affected zones to removing the womb altogether (hysterectomy).

S.O.S.
Period pain

Since this entire book is dedicated to helping you balance your hormones, all its various tips and tricks will hopefully help you make peace with your periods. However, because it is unfortunately one of the most frequent issues keeping women from feeling at ease in their feminine body, I will summarise here some advice to prevent excessive period pain (scientific term: dysmenorrhoea) and regulate your monthly cycles:
◦ Move the pelvis and stretch the psoas and lower back daily, especially during the week before your period. Practise yoga, dance, walk, take the stairs…
◦ Rest more often and compensate stress (relaxation postures, deep breathing).
◦ See a specialist in acupuncture, homeopathy or Ayurveda, or an osteopath – all these methods have proven to be effective for this issue. Herbal remedies have also been used for many centuries, ask a trained herbalist for advice.
◦ Increase your magnesium levels with foot baths or supplements.
◦ Practice the belly massage.
◦ Improve your digestion, so that your body can take up the nutrients it needs in order to balance your hormones.
◦ Keep your lower belly and lower back warm by wearing a *haramaki* or a *Belly Blanket*.
◦ Schedule some moments to be alone, and some moments to connect with other women, so that you can be aware of your needs and desires, and feel supported.

Yoga sequence for ovaries and womb

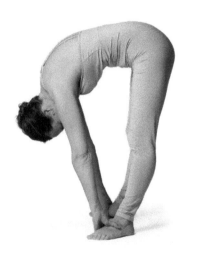

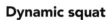

Dynamic squat
(*avoid postnatally, go easy if you are pregnant, skip if the placenta is under the baby*).
Start from a squatting position (see sequence for digestion), but place your hands under your feet (if possible) coming from the inside. Inhale looking forward, and as you exhale, bow your head and lift your hips to come into a standing forward fold, if possible with your hands still under your feet (or else on your calves). Keep your knees slightly bent, especially if your lower back is sensitive. You can straighten the legs completely if your lower back is strong. As you inhale again, return to the squat. Alternate several times between both positions, in a rather dynamic way, breathing strongly through the nose. You can increase your repetitions as you become more familiar with this exercise. End by staying several breaths in a standing forward fold, letting your arms dangle, then bend your knees and come up to standing with a straight back, firmly pushing your feet into the floor.

Hip rotations.
Standing with your feet approximately hip width apart, with soft knees, place your hands on your hips and shift your hips to one side, then stick out your bum backwards, then shift your hips to the other side, and then tilt your tailbone forward. Keep going in a fluid way to create circular motions, starting with small circles and opening up in a spiralling way towards bigger and bigger circles. Then rotate in the opposite direction and start spiralling back from the big circles to smaller and smaller ones. You can also balance from side to side by simply bending one knee, then the other, avoiding any jerky movements keeping your moves fluid and even playful. You can also lift your arms and stretch them up, alternating left and right, whilst you move your hips. Why not put on some music that makes you want to dance, anything goes to keep you moving your hips in this circular, free and playful way for several minutes. (Pregnant women: this can also be a great movement for active labour).

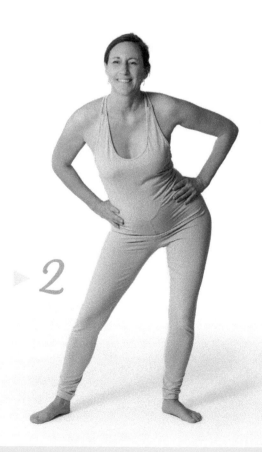

2

Downward-facing dog.
From a standing posture, bend your knees and bow down until your hands touch the ground. Walk your feet back and bring your knees to the ground to be on all fours. As we did in the first sequence, lift both knees off the floor at the same time on an exhalation. Your hips move back and upwards at the same time. Keep your knees slightly bent to really lengthen your back. You could lift one heel, then the other, walking on the spot, to stretch your calf muscles, then after a while, stabilise your posture, staying still. It doesn't matter if your heels don't touch the floor. Keep your ears between your arms. Imagine pushing the floor away with your hands as you breathe deeply. When your arms get tired, come back to all fours.

3

Sphinx. X!
From all fours, bring your elbows and forearms to the floor, elbows more or less under your shoulders, hands flat on the floor, fingers pointing forwards. Bring your pelvis and legs to rest on the floor, toes pointing backwards. You may enjoy padding the floor with a blanket under your belly and hip bones. If your lower back is uncomfortable, engage your glute muscles and bring your heels together, otherwise let the legs relax completely. Keep your ears away from your shoulders, the neck long but tension-free and look forward. Breathe deeply and feel how this creates a belly massage against the floor. Feel how your lower back lifts on the inhalation and sinks down on the exhalation. Stay for as long as you wish. This yin yoga posture works by being held over a longer period of time. To come out of it, bring your hands under your shoulders and return to all fours.

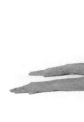

4

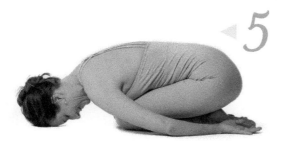

5

Child's pose *(in pregnancy, separate your knees to make space for the belly).*
From all fours, stretch back and bring your buttocks towards your heels. You may want more padding with a blanket or cushion on your heels. Bring your forehead to the floor; or if that's not happening, make fists with your hands and rest your forehead on your stacked fists. Stay in this folded position and feel how your lower back gently stretches. Breathe deeply and slowly. To come out, slowly unfurl your back until you are sitting on your heels.

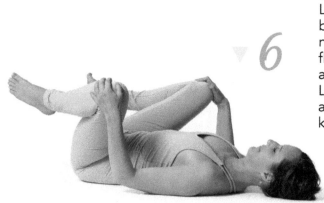

Supine knee circles. X!

Lie down on your back, knees bent, feet on the floor. If needed, place a blanket or flat cushion under head and a blanket under your hips. Lift your feet off the floor and place one hand on each knee. Keeping the hands on the knees, separate your legs and start making circles (knees coming closer to each other and then separating again). Do six repetitions this way, then six rotating in the opposite direction. End by bringing your feet back on the floor.

Half butterfly with raised hip. X!

Comfortably lying on your back, knees bent, feet flat on the floor, touching each other. Open your right knee down to the floor, place a cushion under the knee if that's more comfortable. Rub your palms together to create some heat and place your right hand flat on your right ovary (low on the right side of the belly, in the groin). Extend your left arm behind you on the floor. On an inhalation, lift your left hip just a little off the floor and stretch your left arm further back, you may feel a stretch in the groin. The right hip stays on the floor. On the exhalation, bring the left hip down again. Start with three repetitions per session, and expand to six, then up to twelve as you become more familiar with this movement. Then bring the right knee up again, take a breath to compare the sensations on the left and the right, and change sides by bringing the left knee down, right arm stretched back, for the same number of repetitions. To end, hug your knees into your chest.

Happy baby (pregnancy: maximum until week 30, and go easy).

Lying on your back, knees lifted. With knees still bent, lift the soles of your feet to face the ceiling. Bring your arms between your legs and grab hold of the outer edge of each foot from the inside (for some women it is more convenient to hold the insides of the feet by turning their wrists). The arms start gently pulling on the feet as if you could bring your knees towards the ground on each side of your chest, meanwhile the feet resist. Stay for at least three deep breaths, up to three minutes if you wish. Try to keep your lower back on the floor if possible. In this position you can also roll from side to side if you wish, which can be a nice way to massage out the back. To end the posture, hug your knees to your chest (sideways if pregnant).

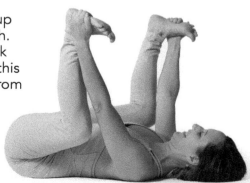

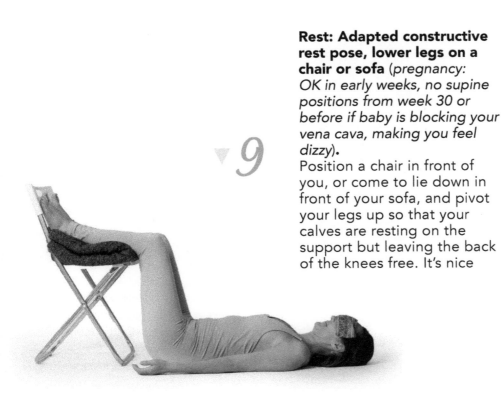

Rest: Adapted constructive rest pose, lower legs on a chair or sofa (*pregnancy: OK in early weeks, no supine positions from week 30 or before if baby is blocking your vena cava, making you feel dizzy*).

▼ *9*

Position a chair in front of you, or come to lie down in front of your sofa, and pivot your legs up so that your calves are resting on the support but leaving the back of the knees free. It's nice to put a blanket under the hips and a flat cushion under the head. Make sure you are warm enough to rest here for several minutes, with your back flat on the floor. Breathe deeply and slowly. Don't rush to come out. Start by bringing the knees towards the chest, then pivot to one side, resting your head on your lower arm, stay several breaths, then use your hands to help you up to a seated position.

MEDITATION
Heart to Womb Mudra

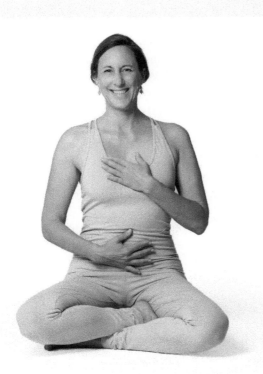

Comfortably seated, back upright, shoulders relaxed. I rub my palms to create warmth. I place my left hand on the centre of my chest, my right hand on my lower belly, between the navel and the pubic bone. I breathe slowly and deeply. With every exhalation I feel my belly gently drawing back towards my spine, with every inhalation the belly relaxes. With my next exhalation I focus on (or imagine) warmth under the hand which is on my belly, and as the inhalation begins, I imagine the warmth travelling upwards, towards the hand on my chest. As I exhale, the warmth travels back down to the belly, and so forth. I can keep going for as long as I like. (… Pause…) When I feel like emerging from this meditation, I can end by chanting three "Om", or visualise a positive image, repeat a positive word, or just smile.

THE WOMB BLESSING

by Nadège Lanvin

Where does the womb blessing come from, and what is it?

Miranda Gray has written books about womanhood, as well as being a healer who has been working with feminine archetypes for over 20 years. In 2011, she created the Womb Blessing. This is an energy healing technique which allows you to connect with the sacred feminine, to reconnect with your authentic feminine nature. The womb blessing is for every woman.

Some women receive the blessing with a specific reason in mind: to repair their womb after illness or aggression, to prepare for in-vitro-fertilisation, to receive a baby, to celebrate it and mark the occasion of a change in their cycle, whilst others simply come to connect with the creative space that is their womb.

Men can also receive a gift, to reconnect with the Divine Feminine and their feminine aspect.

There are Worldwide Womb Blessings five times a year, coinciding with the full moon in February, May, August, October, and December. Over 60 000 women worldwide connect with Miranda Gray and the other women's circles on these occasions, for a meditative and energetic practice (there are 4 time slots over the course of the day to suit different time zones).

You can sign up on Miranda Gray's website: wombblessing.com (translated into every language!) to receive the energy of this worldwide blessing and/ or to take part in a circle organised by a Moon Mother for this occasion.

A Moon Mother is a person who was initiated by Miranda Gray to share these specific healing therapies. The initiation stretches over a few days, during which Miranda Gray explains the technique in detail and gives each participant the opportunity to transmit this energy of the divine Feminine to other women or men. There are several levels of initiation. The www.wombblessing.com website lists all the initiated Moon Mothers worldwide.

You can arrange to meet with a Moon Mother anytime you like to receive the blessing in person and /or an additional energetic treatment.

What happens exactly?

This is how the session is organised:

◦ You will be asked to bring 2 bowls, which will symbolise your womb. A candle will be lit in one of them (the fire, creative symbol of the womb) and water will be poured into the other (the womb being a "watery" environment).

◦ You sit on a chair and the Moon Mother reads the meditation text of the womb blessing.

◦ The Moon Mother gives the blessing by placing her hands on specific areas of your body (including above your head, at the heart level, on the womb, thereby reconnecting you with the energy of the Divine Feminine.

◦ After the blessing, you will either drink the water from your bowl and share it with the Moon Mother (and have a bite to eat), or the Moon Mother will suggest an additional treatment, which you will lie down on the padded floor for.

◦ During the treatment, the Moon Mother reconnects you with the Divine Feminine through 3 "gates": the womb space (the feminine archetypes), the heart region (love), the head (the 'qualities').

◦ After the treatment, you will drink the water from your bowl and share it with the Moon Mother.

The blessing is a very powerful technique, even if you may not feel much to begin with. It may modify your cycle slightly for a month. This is why you need to be careful if you are using a natural contraceptive method. This is also why you should not have more than one blessing per cycle.

The treatment is less powerful than the blessing and can be received as often as you wish. You need not wait for a full moon to receive a womb blessing.

Underneath the womb and the cervix is the vagina, which the penis enters during heterosexual sex, and through which blood flows down during menstruation. When a woman experiences an orgasm, the muscles of the vagina, which are like rings, spontaneously produce rhythmic movements, which can feel like undulations. In the context of procreation, this helps send the sperm upwards towards the cervix.

Outside of this context, these undulations are simply very pleasant. Specific practices to tone the pelvic floor also include the vagina. Some forms of Tantra teach how to voluntarily create these orgasmic undulations (alone or with a partner).

The vagina "self-cleans" throughout the menstrual cycle. The vaginal secretions, whose quantity varies from woman to woman, are produced by glands situated at the cervix level and in the vaginal walls. **The vaginal flora, just like the gut flora, is composed of bacteria which protect the vagina from infections thanks to the acidity they produce**. If the vaginal discharge has an unusual smell or colour, see your gynaecologist to check for a yeast infection or sexually transmitted disease.

Vaginal yeast infections (thrush, mycosis)

Having a healthy vaginal flora is as important as having a healthy gut flora (they often go together) because it prevents vaginal dryness and infections. The vagina's natural pH can be altered by excessive vaginal hygiene or by using soap.

An overly acidic vagina and an imbalance in the vaginal flora will cause certain types of yeast to multiply (mycosis), quite often the ill-famed *candida albicans*, which is naturally present in the body, but causes a problem if it proliferates and becomes a vaginal candidiasis.

Hormonal fluctuations during and after pregnancy, diabetes, endocrine disorders, antibiotics, too much sugar, a gut disorder, wearing overly tight and synthetic clothing, as well as daily use of panty liners, can all cause fungal proliferation. The mycosis could also come from external contamination, from a sexual contact or an object.

The main symptoms of vaginal mycosis are an itching in the area of the vulva and the entry of the vagina, thick white discharge (odourless), a burning sensation and / or a red and swollen vulva. Your GP or gynaecologist can advise about a vaginal suppository (some are prescription-free). It will also be helpful to replenish the flora with vaginal probiotics (which are sold over the counter and can be taken preventatively a few times a year, if you are prone to these infections).

Sanitary products – spoilt for choice?

In the West, we can currently choose from a list of different products to collect our menstrual blood (provided we have the means to pay, which is an issue): the more widespread ones are tampons, with or without applicator, and single-use sanitary pads. If you are concerned about the environmental impact of these products, you may wish to move away from single use products and instead consider alternatives such as the silicone menstrual cup, re-usable cloth sanitary pads, and period underwear.

A French documentary from 2017 by Audrey Gloaguen, "*Tampon, notre ennemi intime*" (i.e. "The Tampon, our Intimate Enemy"), reminded the general public that tampons can cause toxic shock syndrome (TSS), a lesser-known infection due to the bacteria staphylococcus aureus. It is rare, but very dangerous.

To a lesser degree, it can also happen with menstrual cups. This is why you should change your tampon or empty (and clean) your cup approximately every 4 hours.

Apart from the risk of TSS and the pollution aspect, tampons and single-use pads have been targeted by consumer protection agencies, because several toxic chemicals have been found in some brands' products, encouraging those brands to overhaul their ingredients.[xvii]

Apart from their ecological benefit, re-usable products are also cheaper in the long term. For those who don't feel ready to use the cups, re-usable pads and period underwear are worth trying. Both are made of cloth which absorbs the blood, and you rinse the blood out in cold water before putting the product in the washing machine.

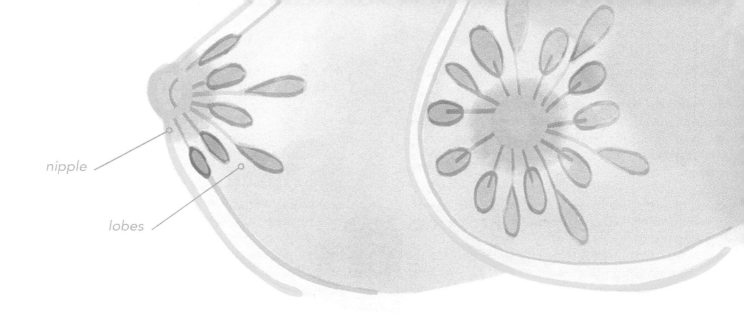

nipple

lobes

Breasts

Breasts are not an organ, but mainly a gland, with two functions: feeding baby, and contributing to a woman's sexual pleasure (and that of her partner!). **The breast is composed of a mammary gland, of supporting ligaments, and of fat**. Their quantity and relative proportion vary from one woman to another. There are also nerves, blood vessels, and lymphatic vessels in the breast. Chains of lymphatic nodes filter out microbes and protect the body from infections and disease. The mammary gland is divided into 15 to 20 sections called "lobes". They are connected with channels which converge at the nipple (situated more or less in the middle of the breast).

In early puberty, hormones (in particular oestrogen) cause an accumulation of fatty tissue under the nipple. The size and shape of the breast will be the result of how these tissues are distributed, not of the gland itself. The cells which will later produce milk in the mammary gland will only become fully active during pregnancy.

The muscles create an erection of the nipple when stimulated sexually or by the feeding baby. Nipple stimulation also stimulates the clitoris and increases the production of prolactin and oxytocin by the pituitary gland.

It is completely normal to have two breasts of different shape or size, some women even have three nipples. The breast size will also change throughout the menstrual cycle as well as during pregnancy. Breasts will also change with age, losing some of their firmness, because the proportion between fatty tissue and fascia will change. Breasts are very sensitive to hormonal fluctuations. Water retention in the second half of the cycle can cause a feeling of swelling or inflammation, which is benign, but can be uncomfortable. Prostaglandins and cytokines, which also cause menstrual cramps, are responsible for this swelling. When hormonal balance is restored, these issues tend to improve or disappear. The changes your breasts undergo during the menstrual cycle mirror those of the womb, with one big difference: the fluid and tissue accumulated in the uterus are then expelled with the next period, whereas those of the breasts are reabsorbed by the body. Lumps or benign knots often disappear by themselves. Cysts (round pockets with liquid inside) are frequent in perimenopause, due to hormonal fluctuations, and they mostly disappear after menopause. If in doubt, always consult your family doctor or gynaecologist. All women really should know their breasts well, and check them regularly to detect any changes early on, a good habit to develop and keep throughout your life. Whilst most changes are harmless, the sooner anything more serious is discovered and treated, the higher the chances to heal completely.

I learned the basics of this technique in my ayurvedic massage training. The Chinese tradition of Taoism has a similar practice. You'll find a (clothed) demonstration of it on my Youtube channel.

This massage is both pleasant and useful – the sensations are pleasant, and at the same time we check on the state of our breasts to detect changes. **Some women say that regular practice helps with premenstrual syndrome and uncomfortable swelling** (like a lymphatic drainage), some also claim it makes their breasts fuller, or even enhances their libido.
Whilst there are many types of specially designed creams, a neutral massage oil (of great quality please, no endocrine disruptors!) will do the trick. Ayurveda considers coconut oil to be cooling and sesame oil to be rather neutral. For swollen breasts, try the castor oil mentioned for the belly massage, since it has anti-inflammatory properties, however it is sticky, so mix it with another oil for your fingers to glide more easily. Go easy, especially if your breasts hurt. Some women find this more practical to do lying down on the bed, or whilst having a bath.

Wash your hands in warm water. Drip a bit of oil into the palm of one hand and then heat it by rubbing your palms. Add more oil as you go along, to ensure easy gliding of your fingers on the skin.

1) Left hand under the right breast, thumb between the breasts, the other fingers on the outer side of the right breast. Make an upward movement of the hand, lifting the breast along, whilst the thumb comes closer to the other fingers, meeting them at the nipple, which you then seize and gently stretch forward. Repeat as often as you like, then change sides.

2) Lift the left hand and place it behind your head to open up the armpit. With your right hand, trace a figure 8 lying on its side (or call it a butterfly) three times around both breasts by crossing your path in the middle and really going all the way up into the armpit. Make sure to caress the entire surface of the breast and armpit, to really feel the structure of the flesh under the skin. Change hands and repeat three times towards the other armpit.

Practice this massage as often as you like. To check on your breast health, the best time is just after your period, when the breasts are least swollen.

"Intimacy": pelvic floor, vulva, and clitoris

For many women, even though they may well be sexually active, their pelvic floor and vulva are *terra incognita*, a mysterious part of their anatomy, until life "forces them" to take a closer look, for instance when they give birth, suffer from incontinence, or have frequent urinary tract infections (UTI).

This part of the female body has long been taboo, and some cultures still mutilate girls' genitals today. This is a real health hazard which also affects a woman's sexuality.

Luckily, mentalities are changing, at least in the West. Some celebrities now even openly advocate using jade eggs, geisha balls, and vaginal steaming.

So let's discover our intimacy, and I encourage you to find a place to be alone for a while, grab a mirror, and have a proper look.

Pelvic floor

The perineum or pelvic floor is actually a group of muscles and ligaments, interwoven to create a "hammock" structure at the bottom of the pelvis, between the legs. Its borders are the pubic symphysis at the front, the sitting bones on the sides, and the tip of the tailbone or coccyx at the back.

The muscles form different "layers" (superficial, middle, deep). The deepest layer is the pelvic diaphragm, shaped like a dome. The next level holds the deep transverse perineal muscle, which connects the two sides of the pelvis, and the urethra (a small sphincter that our urine passes through). The superficial level, composed of 4 muscles and of the external anal sphincter, surrounds the three openings (urethra, vagina, and anus) forming a figure of 8, connecting the front and back of the pelvis. The anal sphincter is the thickest part of the female pelvic floor and often easier to feel and mobilise than the vagina and urethra, so this is a good place to start when you begin practicing pelvic floor exercises to improve its elasticity.

As you can see in the drawing, the pelvic floor is connected to the gluteus muscles (buttocks) and to the adductors (muscles on the inside of the thighs). You may sometimes think you are moving your pelvic floor when you are actually activating the glutes, so you need to learn to feel the difference, touching and looking if necessary. This is also why **strong legs and glutes will influence the tone and blood flow in the pelvic floor area**.

There are many blood vessels and nerves in the pelvic floor, which makes it very sensitive. Staying seated on a chair for too long will slow down blood and lymphatic circulation, which in Eastern medicine traditions is called "stagnation".

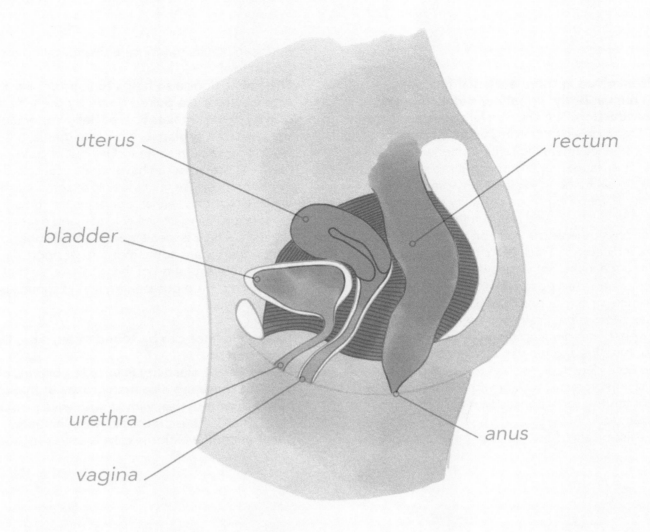

uterus

rectum

bladder

urethra

anus

vagina

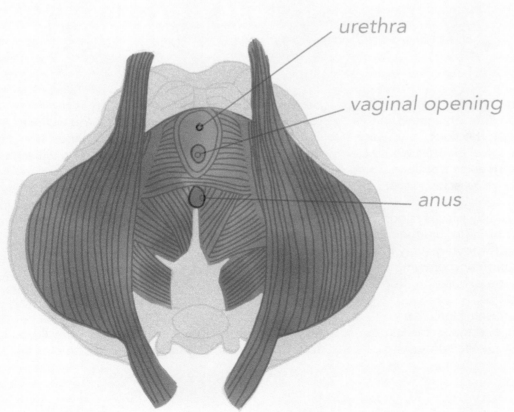

urethra

vaginal opening

anus

It is involved in three essential functions of the human body: urination, defecation and reproduction. The first two functions explain why an elastic pelvic floor is important to prevent or heal incontinence (meaning urine or faeces leaks when sneezing, laughing, or running/jumping).

The sexual function explains why practitioners of some forms of Tantra (who use sexuality to "raise" their level of consciousness) and also sex therapists and pelvic floor physiotherapists insist on toning it if it lacks tone. One indicator of a lack of tone in these muscles, apart from urine leaks, are vaginal "farts" (in yoga, they can occur in inverted postures) and the weakness, or even absence, of sensations during sexual intercourse.

It has been scientifically proven, most famously by Dr Kegel, that developing more tone in the pelvic floor muscles and the vagina can help many women who considered themselves to be "frigid" experience satisfying orgasms, with or without a partner, and to heighten the sensations for a male partner during penetration.[xviii]

An elastic pelvic floor can also help to empty the Bartholin glands to lubricate the vulva and the vagina (see below).

The pelvic floor also helps to support our internal organs which are pulled down by the effects of gravity, which makes it especially important in the case of a prolapse, when the uterus, urethra, bladder or rectum seem to "fall out of position", or "sink". A prolapse can have various causes: difficult births, menopause (all tissues lose some elasticity with falling oestrogen levels), operations in the abdomen, inadequate lifting of heavy loads, and excessive standing. There is also a genetic predisposition. Giving the organs some muscular support helps to stabilise the evolution of the prolapse, so that an operation can be postponed, and in some cases even avoided.

The pelvic floor can be toned at any age, like any other muscle.

The notion of elasticity is very important, however, because there are also many cases of hypertonic pelvic floor muscles, with an excessive involuntary contraction of these muscles, which hinders penetration (the extreme case is called vaginismus).

THE "PELVIC FLOOR BREATH"

An exercise for pelvic floor elasticity (for sexual pleasure, vaginal lubrication, incontinence, postnatal rehabilitation)

Sit on the floor in a kneeling position, on a bolster or several cushions, or on a chair (in this case keep your feet flat on the floor). If you are new at this, rolling up a towel (heated would be even better!), placed lengthwise between your legs, might help to feel the muscles move.

Breathe deeply, and begin by placing your hands flat on your lower ribcage, one hand on each side. Feel your hands moving away from each other on the inhalation and drawing in closer to each other on the exhalation. Repeat until it becomes easy to do.

Now add your buttock muscles into this exercise: when you exhale, engage the glutes as if you were trying to squeeze something between your buttock cheeks (such as the rolled-up towel if you are using it). You will rise slightly higher on your seat, but not lift off it. Relax the muscles on the inhalation (you will sink down slightly). Repeat several times.

You will probably feel the **muscles of your lower belly**, between the pubic bone and the navel, drawing slightly inwards when you exhale and squeeze your butt cheeks together. Now deepen and extend this movement towards the muscles between your legs, your pelvic floor. Feel your **anus** closing and drawing up into your body a little when you exhale. On the inhalation, relax slowly and fully. As you become more experienced, you will be able to feel your **vagina**, which can also close

In such cases you will focus on relaxing the muscles, and seeing a specialised therapist to address both the physical and the psychological aspects will be particularly helpful.

What affects the pelvic floor?

Many things can put pressure on the pelvic floor: baby's weight during pregnancy, vaginal births, repeated and strong sneezing or coughing, slouching on sofas and chairs (which pushes the internal organs down), obesity, forgetting to bend the knees when lifting heavy loads, chronic constipation (worsened by modern toilets, on which we sit as on a chair, instead of squatting) and inappropriate abdominal exercises (crunches and sit-ups in particular).

As mentioned above, menopause, with its adverse effect on tissue elasticity, also affects the tone of the pelvic floor.

How to help your pelvic floor?

○ Practice specific movements to either tone or relax it (see box), especially around pregnancy and in perimenopause. For pregnant women, a targeted auto-massage for the pelvic floor from week 36 onwards can also help prevent tearing during labour (ask your midwife for details).
○ If you practice abdominal exercises, choose the so-called "hypopressive" type.
○ Find a way to elevate your feet when you sit on the toilet so as to resemble more of a squatting posture.
○ When you lift heavy loads, bend your knees, engage the pelvic floor muscles, draw your navel in and up (this way you avoid your internal organs being pressed down).
○ Walk without shoes if possible (with thick socks on cold floors), tone your feet and avoid high heels, because a toned pelvic floor begins with toned feet (especially avoid dropping the arches of the feet too much, as in "flat feet").
○ Tone your adductor muscles (inner thighs) and glutes, as well as your psoas, this muscle which connects the upper and lower body and runs through the pelvis (see box "unsung heroes" in the last chapter).

and draw upwards on the exhalation, and relax on the inhalation, with the urethra and clitoris just following along. Your lower abdominal muscles accompany this movement, which is uninterrupted, like waves coming and going. Once you are quite familiar with this exercise, focus less on the glutes and much more on the anus and the vagina.
Keep breathing deeply and using this technique until you can really feel that your breath is initiated in the pelvic floor, which takes part in its rhythm just like your thoracic diaphragm (the large dome-shaped muscle between your lungs and your belly, which we saw towards the beginning of the book). The exhalation begins at the vagina and the anus, both are drawn up, the belly draws inwards, the ribs draw towards each other, the air eventually comes out of the nostrils.
Both movements are important, the closing and lifting just as much as the relaxing. **What we are looking for is elasticity of these muscles.** Those of you who feel that they need to tone their pelvic floor will extend the exhalation, those who know that they are rather too contracted in this area will focus on letting go when they inhale.
There is no need for geisha balls or jade eggs, and you can do this anytime, anywhere, which is rather handy, as it's "invisible yoga"! It can also be quite enjoyable!

Important: for pregnant women, this technique is practiced with an open-mouthed exhalation, and **"in reverse"**, because the aim in pregnancy is to **prepare the body to open during labour**. So in this case: on the **inhalation engage the muscles, on the exhalation relax them** and imagine your vagina opening like a blossoming flower. Lengthen the exhalation for as long as you comfortably can, never hold your breath when you are pregnant.

The vulva

The vulva is one of these intimate body parts many women are not familiar with. Some current online projects such as *The Vulva Gallery*, which combines drawings of multi-coloured vulvas and sexual education, contribute to making women more comfortable in their bodies, so that they no longer feel the pressure to conform to a norm which actually does not exist. Some women actually undergo elective surgery to change the aspect of this ultra-sensitive body part.

Every woman is different – some have inner labia or lips which are bigger than the outer ones. They can be of different sizes on the left and right. The clitoris also varies in size.

The vulva is in the anterior half of the pelvic floor.

The *labia majora* or outer lips surround the opening of the vagina (sometimes called the vestibule) and the *labia minora* or inner lips, as well as the clitoris. During puberty, under the influence of sexual hormones, hair starts growing on the pubis. The vulva also gradually changes, two to three years before the first period: the labia develop, the vulval opening becomes horizontal, and the clitoris grows in size.

Some women have a lot of pubic hair on their labia majora, some have little. It is obviously your personal choice whether to let this hair grow or remove it, however know that they are a natural protection of the skin of the outer lips and help to keep the level of humidity just right.

Inside the *labia majora* are the *labia minora*, sometimes also called "nymphs".

The *labia minora* meet to form the hood of the **clitoris**, an erectile part which has a glans at its tip.

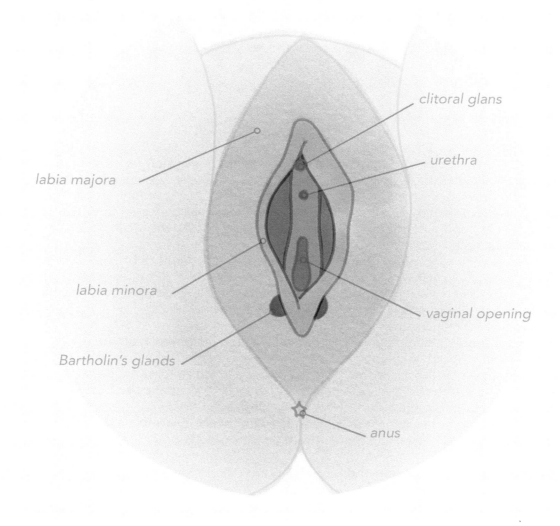

labia majora

labia minora

Bartholin's glands

clitoral glans

urethra

vaginal opening

anus

80

The glans is the only visible part of the clitoris, which also features two bulbs and two roots, which surround the entrance of the vagina. Vaginal sexual stimulation is therefore simply stimulation of a different part of the clitoris. The glans swells and emerges from its hood when sexually excited, just like that male penis.

French researcher Odile Fillod created a 3-D-printable, creative commons-licensed, clitoris model. It is currently contributing to transforming sexual education on the topic of an organ which had actually almost disappeared from anatomy manuals. Apparently, this was due to the fact that the clitoris is the only organ which only has one function: the woman's sexual pleasure. (https://odilefillod.wixsite.com/clitoris).

Under the clitoris are the **urethra, the paraurethral glands** (or Skene glands, this is where female ejaculation happens), the opening of the **vagina**, partly covered by the hymen in virgins, and the **Bartholin glands**, which help to lubricate the vagina during intercourse by secreting a transparent mucus. These glands are usually invisible and they atrophy after menopause, which is one of the reasons why women after menopause can suffer from vaginal dryness. Lubricants can then help make intercourse more comfortable.
The Hormone Yoga method developed by Dinah Rodrigues, which raises the levels of oestrogen, is proven to help with vaginal dryness. The pelvic floor breathing method presented above is also helpful.

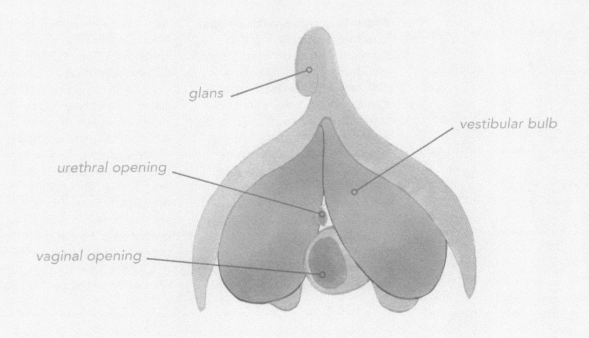

glans

vestibular bulb

urethral opening

vaginal opening

Yoga sequence
for the pelvic floor

Shake it out.
Have fun shaking yourself out like a wet dog, shaking out your whole body, from your fingertips to your buttocks and your face, bouncing up and down. Blow "raspberries" making a "brrrr" sound with your lips as you exhale through the mouth. Claim your space, let it all go, keep shaking for as long as you like, for at least one minute! Then stand still, arms hanging down, and enjoy the sensation of having sparkling "bubbles" inside your body, feeling alive.

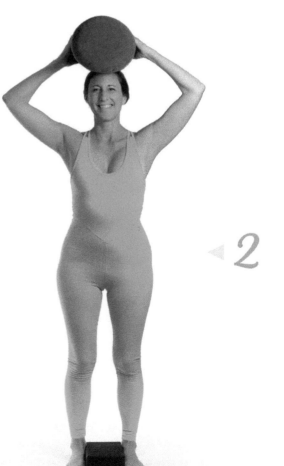

Mountain pose with props.
You need something a bit heavy to carry on your head (I am demonstrating with a yoga bolster) and something you can squeeze between your feet (like a yoga brick), so that your feet are approximately hip width apart. Standing up begin by lifting all your toes off the floor, then bring them back down and really push them firmly back down, especially the big toe, for a strong base and lifted inner arches of the feet. Squeeze the object between your feet, feel yourself rooted in the floor and with active inner thigh muscles. Place the heavy object on your head and hold it up there with both hands. Feel how pushing your head upwards against the object makes you stand taller, more upright. The whole body is well placed, long and active, the pelvic floor is engaged. Stay this way for at least one minute and really endeavour to create a body memory, so that over time you will know how to stand in this way even without the props.

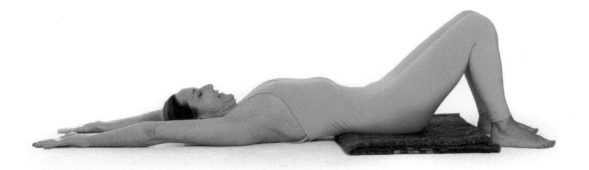

Constructive rest pose with abdominal lock. X!

Lie on your back, with a blanket under the hips and buttocks, support your head too, if needed. Knees bent, feet on the floor, hip distance apart, adjust the position of your feet closer or further away from your buttocks, so that you feel at ease and your lower back has no more than its slight natural curve. Stretch your arms over head and interlace your fingers, really lengthen your upper body. Breathe deeply and slowly. With each exhalation, press your lower back into the floor and tuck your navel in towards your spine to create a hollow in your belly and a sensation of vacuum. Engage the pelvic floor muscles by closing the anus and the vaginal opening. Stay a few seconds with 'empty lungs' if possible. When you feel the need to inhale, release the belly and pelvic floor, and the natural curvature returns in your lower back as your pelvic tilt changes. Repeat a total of three times. Then relax your arms and legs on the floor.

Active bridge (pregnancy: only in the first trimester or until your belly starts protruding).

Lying on your back, arms alongside the body, knees bent, feet on the floor, heels close to the buttocks, place a firm cushion or yoga brick between your thighs and squeeze it. On an exhalation, lift your buttocks off the floor, then your lower back, then your middle back. The bodyweight shifts towards the shoulders. Feet stay on the floor, keep squeezing the object between your thighs. Inhale when you have reached your highest position. As you exhale, draw your navel in towards your spine, engage the pelvic floor, and slowly unfurl your back little by little unto the floor. Repeat six times at your own pace, take extra breaths in between if needed.

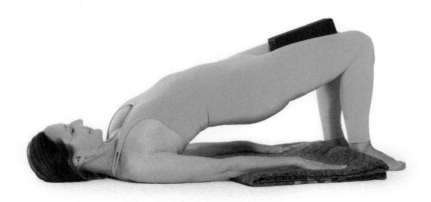

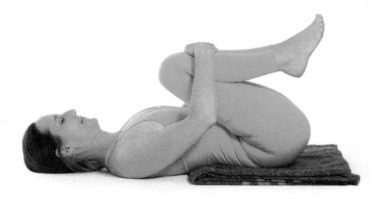

5 Knees to chest pose

(pregnancy: legs apart to make space for baby, and only until week 30).
Lying on your back, hug your knees in towards your chest. Draw them closer on the exhalation and release the knees away a little on the inhalation. You could also roll from side to side in this position, which can be very nice for the lower back. Stay as long as you like.

6 Rest: Supported butterfly pose (aka "resting queen")

(Postnatal: legs extended instead of butterfly pose).
Create a stable and comfortable support, sloping down, with pillows, bricks if available, and a bolster on top, lengthwise. Place a folded blanket in front of the end of the bolster which is touching the floor, and sit on the blanket. You may want to add pillows under your open knees and maybe some extra support under your head if it tilts too far back once you lie on the bolster. Knees bent up, feet on the floor, recline on the bolster and check the height is right for you, and if not, add or remove some pillows until you feel fully comfortable. You want to avoid exacerbating the curve in your lower back to a point of discomfort. Once the back is settled, open your knees, soles of the feet touching, into a butterfly shape. The closer your feet are to your buttocks, the deeper the stretch will be in the inner thighs, so glide the feet a bit further down if needed. It can be really nice to have a blanket, pillow, or hot water bottle on your belly as you lie in this position. Stay for at least five minutes. To exit the posture, bring your knees together, put your hands flat on the floor, tuck your chin in, and use your arms and abdominal muscles to help you sit up.

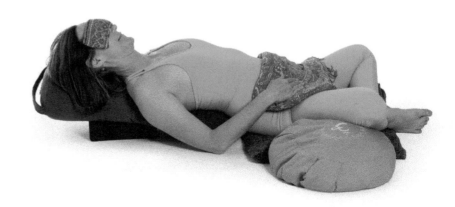

MEDITATION
Blossoming Flower Mudra

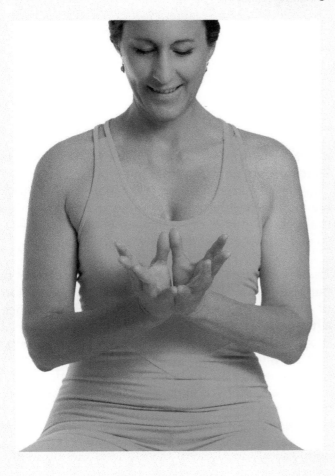

Comfortably seated, back upright, shoulders relaxed, I bring my hands together in front of my chest, heels of the hands and tips of the fingers touching, but keeping a hollow space between the palms, as if I were protecting something delicate with my hands. I now imagine that my hands are a flower bud about to blossom. Traditionally it is meant to be a lotus, but a rose or any favourite flower is fine. I inhale through the nose, and as I exhale, I softly blow on my closed fingertips. Thumbs and pinkie fingers of both hands stay together in pairs, but the other six fingers slowly start to separate like petals of a blooming flower. I inhale again, and on the exhalation I blow on my fingers again, so they open some more. And so forth until my hands are a wide open flower, beautiful and radiant, I smile at it and behold it, and when I feel ready, I lift my arms up and spread my hands, as if to offer this flower to the world around me. I softly place my hands back on my thighs and stay like this in contemplation for as long as I like.

Women's Circles

Where do they come from?

Several cultural and religious traditions, from the Aborigines to Judaism to the people of Tibet, had separate spaces for women during their menstruation, due to taboos which saw them as "impure" during this time. Being isolated in this way, sometimes in precarious circumstances, could be difficult, yet in other contexts, these times apart from the rest of the group were considered a rite of passage, an initiation, during which the ancestral wisdom was passed on by older women - or just a break from the family and the tribe.

Independently of their periods, women often worked or worshipped amongst themselves and would chat or sing at the same time, such as the American pioneer women who would gather for a "quilting bee" to help each other finish their patchwork bed covers.

What's in it for you?

Learning, sharing, ritual, solidarity and sisterhood – these are the aspects which interest and fascinate today's women who create groups with names including "red tent", "moon circle" or "life circle". These groups can bring together women of different social backgrounds and various ages around all sorts of issues.

The Womb Blessing, which Nadège Lanvin described earlier, is an example of a women's circle which meets on the full moon.

The simple fact of meeting in a cheerful spirit and feeling heard without judgement can often be enough to lighten our load, or to find within ourselves the solution to whatever may be worrying us.

These meetings have proven beneficial effects on our emotional wellbeing, thanks to the secretion of oxytocin by the pituitary gland. This substance, a hormone as well as a neurotransmitter, is better known for its influence on the womb muscles during and just after childbirth, as well as on the mammary glands (and the baby's brain) during breastfeeding. In these situations, it encourages bonding between mother and child. Oxytocin also helps bonding between romantic partners, creating this connection of tenderness and trust which often overtakes sexual attraction over time.

Apart from maternity and courting, it has been established **that oxytocin also increases trust, empathy and generosity** amongst friends or acquaintances, **whilst reducing stress and anxiety.**[xix]

How does it work?

Each group chooses its format and establishes its own rules – confidentiality and kindness are always amongst them. Choosing a welcoming location and adding a bit of decoration, such as flowers, candles and comfortable cushions, helps to create the right atmosphere. A theme may be defined beforehand, maybe with the suggestion of sharing a poem, text or song that reflects it. Obviously, you may also choose to meet simply to enjoy a specific activity together and keep some time at the end to relax around a cup of tea, in order to share thoughts and feelings.

In some circles, women practise certain techniques to gradually improve the connection with their body and their intuition (sensory experiences, movement or dance, massage, meditation).
There is usually some time reserved for talking. This could involve passing a symbolic object around, signifying that only the woman holding the object is now invited to speak, whilst the others are asked to listen to her without interrupting, commenting or offering advice, which could either happen later or not at all.

Kindness is really an important factor, and if talking time is part of the format, it is useful to make sure that at least one of the facilitators is familiar with the psychological aspects of group work, to make sure that all participants feel heard and respected. Otherwise, some people may monopolise the conversation whilst others hold back, depending on their character.
Whether you join or co-create a group, do watch out, especially at first: observe exactly how you feel just after the session and the next day – it is normal to

feel emotional if the evening touched you deeply, but if you feel uneasy, sad, or picked upon by the group (or they ask you for a hefty sum of money!), this is not the group you need, and you would do well to heed your intuition.

How to use this guide for your circle

Should you wish to use the practises in this book to start a programme for your circle, you could meet to enjoy the physical movements, the breathing techniques, the massages, and the meditations, share your experiences with the practical tips such as the *haramaki* or the foot bath, and discuss the themes presented in the chapters.

If you meet on a weekly basis, you can repeat the postures and exercises of just one chapter over a month to really integrate them and feel their effects taking hold. Then move onto the next chapter for a month. After four months, you will know all the practices well. You can then return to the beginning, and you will realise how much each part also enhances the other ones.
If you meet once a month (which is the most common format, often following the full moon calendar), you will probably choose to do a different practice each time.
If you meet for a full week-end, in a "wellness retreat" format, you could dedicate half a day to each of the chapters.

BEING YIN IN A YANG WORLD

by Mirjam Wagner

Women have an innate ability to adapt and go with the flow. From a very young age, we are exposed to the natural cycles, which simply oblige us to surrender to rhythms that are not under our control.

Through our intense hormonal and emotional changes, we get in touch with nature's law of death and rebirth on a regular basis. We know instinctively when to stand still and surrender or when to gather our energies and move forward. However, our modern world is much more dominated by yang principles. Faster, higher & further are the key words to describe success. We are educated to ignore the strong voices of our intuition and instead follow the strong call for functioning, achieving and stay active. It is not very well regarded, let alone encouraged, to listen to our bodies, to pause, soften and be still. These qualities are much rather related to weakness and failure. It is important for us to understand that finding ways to express our yin aspects is crucial for a healthy balance on a personal and global level. It is essential for us to look for the company of other women where we feel safe and connected to the vital feminine source, the Yin. Once we have re-established our intuitive bond with our yin qualities, we can enjoy the yang sides from a place of serenity and inner strength.

Let's remember that our bodies are a representation of nature's unique beauty and perfection. All our systems, especially the endocrine system, provide us with the necessary elements to grow, to compensate and to heal.

Progesterone and Oestrogen are our sexual hormones and considered the Yin aspect of our body. They are the counterpart of our Yang side, represented by the stress hormones, such as adrenaline and cortisol.

The more Yin hormones are circulating in our body, the better we can cope with stressful situations in our life. Around the age of 35, the production of progesterone starts to decrease. This means that any yang aspect, such as stress, will be experienced much more intensely than before.

Another important drop of oestrogen and progesterone happens at the age of menopause. If at this point we continue with the same habits as when we were 25, our bodies can no longer maintain a healthy balance and we literally collapse, break down, or burn out.

Once we become aware of these natural processes in our inner landscape it will be easier for us to consciously adapt lifestyle, diet and levels of stress. **Acknowledging these important changes allows us to make wise choices, so we can move through the years with ease and grace.**

This book's women's circle

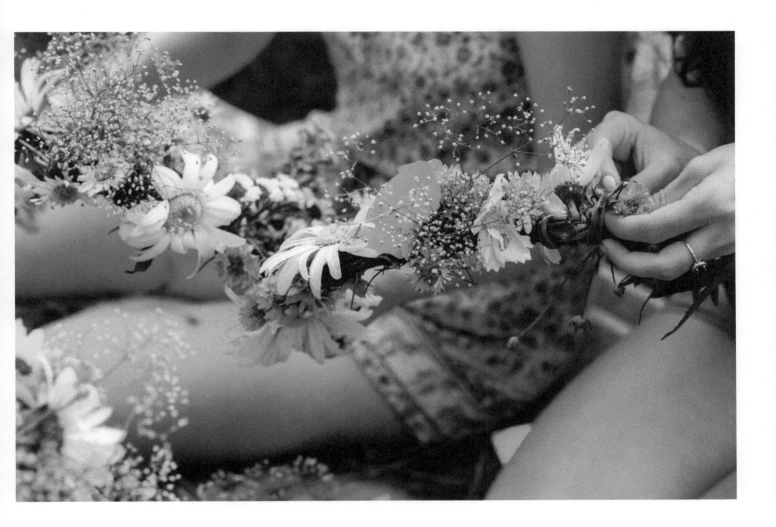

Now is the time to introduce you to our virtual women's circle, this book's co-authors. My dream would be to bring them all together one day, "for real" in the same room – oxytocin levels, energy and belly laughs would probably skyrocket!

I hope their life stories will inspire you to choose experienced and kind practitioners who will guide you on your own path to health and wellbeing. I also hope you will agree that a woman who learns to listen to her body's messages can transform her own life – and often that of others.

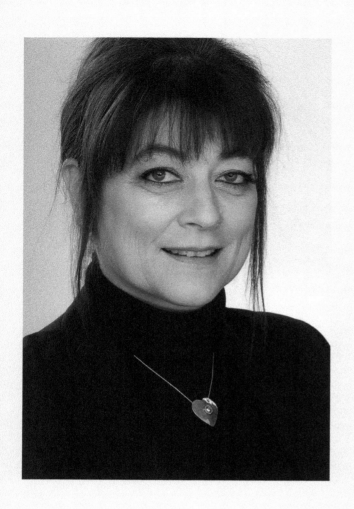

Jani White

Jani White is an internationally renowned lecturer and writer in Chinese medicine for Fertility & Pregnancy. She is an acupuncturist, doula and antenatal teacher with over 29 years' experience of UK maternity and gynaecology services. Jani is the Director of AcuHouse, bringing together a talented network of practitioners providing integrative healthcare.

Jani's specialities are wide ranging, though the core of her work is in one pillar - the Endocrine System - your hormones. She treats all ages, both male and female, infant to geriatric and everyone in between: Fertility & Gynaecology / Pregnancy & Childbirth / Post Natal / Men's Sexual, Reproductive and Uro-genital Health / Prostate / Menopause/ Infants / Children / Teenagers.

Jani is a Senior Lecturer and she teaches extensively in Obstetrics, Gynaecology & Fertility, and Andrology, both nationally and internationally, based from the MA degree program she wrote for Oxford Brookes University. She is the Founder and was Chair of the Acupuncture Fertility Network (AFN) 2006-2014, and she set up and chaired ACT London (Acupuncture for Childbirth Team) 2006-2013.

Jani advocates an integrative approach to treatment, combining the best of both Western and Chinese medicine. Her work is dedicated to providing quality integrative education, emphasising the balance between Safe Practice, Informed Choice and Supportive Care.

When she is not in clinic or busy writing a 5-book series about how our hormones work - the first is called 'The Fertile Fizz' - Jani can be found happily tramping across London's Hampstead Heath in all weathers with her dogs.

For a detailed look at the depth and range of Jani's work please visit:
www.acuhouse.co.uk
www.fertilefizz.com
www.janiwhite.com

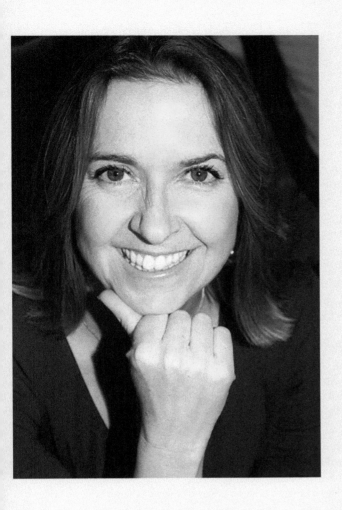

Sarah Davison

It was a long road for Sarah to become a homeopath, but a road well worth travelling. She started out with a degree in Russian, then went into international sales, using her French and Italian instead. Seven years later, with a lot more confidence, but feeling very unfulfilled, she left her job to do a Graduate Diploma in Psychology. She then spent a very happy and fulfilled 14 years as a consultant, trainer and coach to big corporates in the arena of innovation and creativity. She loved this career, which involved a lot of travel, and she was known by her colleagues for always travelling with her portable homeopathy kit - her passion for homeopathy was already evident. The job also required her to train as a Master Practitioner of Neuro-Linguistic Programming (NLP), which she now uses to coach clients.

With the advent of Motherhood at 41 and trying to flexi-work (unsuccessfully), by the time she was 46, perimenopausal hormones meant she could no longer handle the stress like she used to. So she combined her passion for coaching and for homeopathy into a new career. With a Bachelor of Science with first class Honours in Homeopathy, she successfully set up The Coaching Homeopath in London in 2012. She specialises in helping women through the challenges of menopause and has designed an online course.

To find out more, please visit:
www.thrivehomeopathy.com

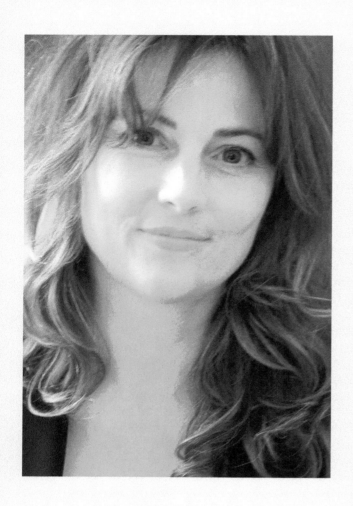

Stéfanie L'olivret

Stéfanie holds a French doctorate in pharmacy and has over twenty years of experience in the health and wellbeing sector. Working directly with patients in pharmacies and hospitals convinced her of the importance of adding another dimension to the conventional therapeutic approach. Her research into the compatibility of modern science and mindfulness techniques connecting the mind and the body brought her to Ayurveda.

She trained with several masters in France, India and the United States, in particular with Vaidya Atreya Smith and Doctor Vasant Lad. Witnessing more and more benefits of Ayurveda in her own life and that of her patients, she then broadened her knowledge base by studying yoga, Ayurveda's sister science.
She spent several months in Indian ashrams, studying integral yoga at the Bihar School of Yoga and Akhanda Yoga in Rishikesh under Yogrishi Vishvketu (RYT 500). She has also sat for several silent meditation retreats (Vipassana).
Firmly believing that Western and Eastern medical systems can work in synergy, Stéfanie now divides her time between clinical pharmacology work and transmitting authentic forms of Ayurveda and yoga with their holistic approach to healing.

She works in France and travels frequently to India, where she organises retreats in French, as well as returning regularly to Rishikesh to teach Ayurveda within the Akhanda Yoga teacher training courses.

www.stefanielolivret.com

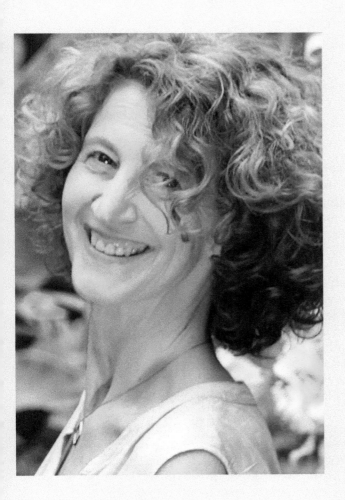

Tiffany Bown

Tiffany's own healing journey - and her interest in natural approaches to women's health and wellbeing - began nearly 20 years ago when she went through a four-year fertility struggle before the birth of her first child. This deeply painful experience was the gift that set her off down the road of healing and discovery and motivated her to train so she could help other women navigate and transform their own life challenges. After studying Chinese at university, she spent 10 years in crazy, polluted, fun Beijing, where she lived in a linear, push-on-through way that destroyed her health, but then discovered the wonders of acupuncture, Chinese herbs, Tuina massage and Yoga. From there she moved to Italy for 11 years, where she had her three children, trained to be a Naturopath and Reflexologist and studied Iyengar Yoga with Gabriela Corsico-Piccolini. She then met MogaDao founder Zhenzan Dao and discovered first MogaDao Yoga and then the beauty and healing power of Qigong. She moved to Cambridge, UK, in 2011 with her family and has continued to study, notably with Birthlight founder Françoise Freedman for fertility, prenatal and Wellwoman yoga, and with Uma Dinsmore-Tuli for Womb Yoga. She is passionate about helping other women to embrace the power of their cyclical feminine reality and to heal and blossom with Yoga and Qigong.

To find out more, please visit:
www.nurtureworksyoga.co.uk

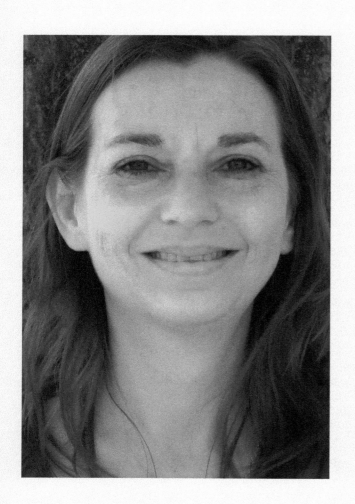

Nadège Lanvin

Born with a light disability, Nadège witnessed yoga's powerful health benefits from a young age. After twenty years of practice, whilst she was working in a photography agency, she decided to retrain and become a professional yoga instructor. She trained with Sivananda for her first yoga teacher training qualification, then with Satyananda in yoga nidra, followed by yoga therapy with the Indian master Saji. She has also trained in hormone yoga with Dinah Rodrigues and became a Moon Mother, initiated by Miranda Gray. In 2012 she opened Yoga and Co, her own yoga studio in the heart of Paris. Her yoga practice is centred around finding alternative, soft, ecological, and joyful solutions to health issues, and to support physical and mental health. This expanded organically into a further career as a writer. She began by contributing articles to Esprit Yoga magazine, and is now the author of several yoga therapy books in French. Her time is currently divided between teaching, writing, and running her yoga studio.

To find out more, please visit:
www.yogaandco.fr

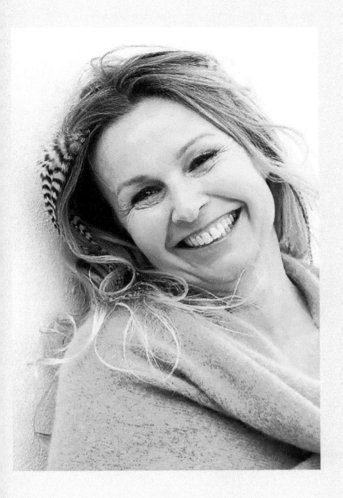

Mirjam Wagner

Mirjam is passionate about her work as an osteopath, yoga teacher, and teacher trainer. When she discovered the tranquil practice of Yin yoga and yoga therapy, she knew she had found her path. She loves working with women to discover conscious and subconscious limitations of their real potential through feminine archetypes and hormones.

In her teaching, Mirjam combines her deep understanding of anatomy with a healing spiritual approach. Sarah Powers, Paul Grilley, Gil Hedley, Ted Kapchuk, doctor Daniel Keown & Jean Bolen are amongst those who most influenced her and inspired her on her path. Her vast experience, as well as her thorough knowledge of the human body closely linked to emotional and mental health allow her to be a very kind and inspiring teacher who will guide you towards a deeper connection with yourself and others.

Based in Palma de Mallorca, she teaches in Europe and Brazil during workshops, retreats and teacher training courses, and also runs her own online yoga studio.

To find out more, including about her book and online course to balance hormones, please visit: www.yogatherapymallorca.com

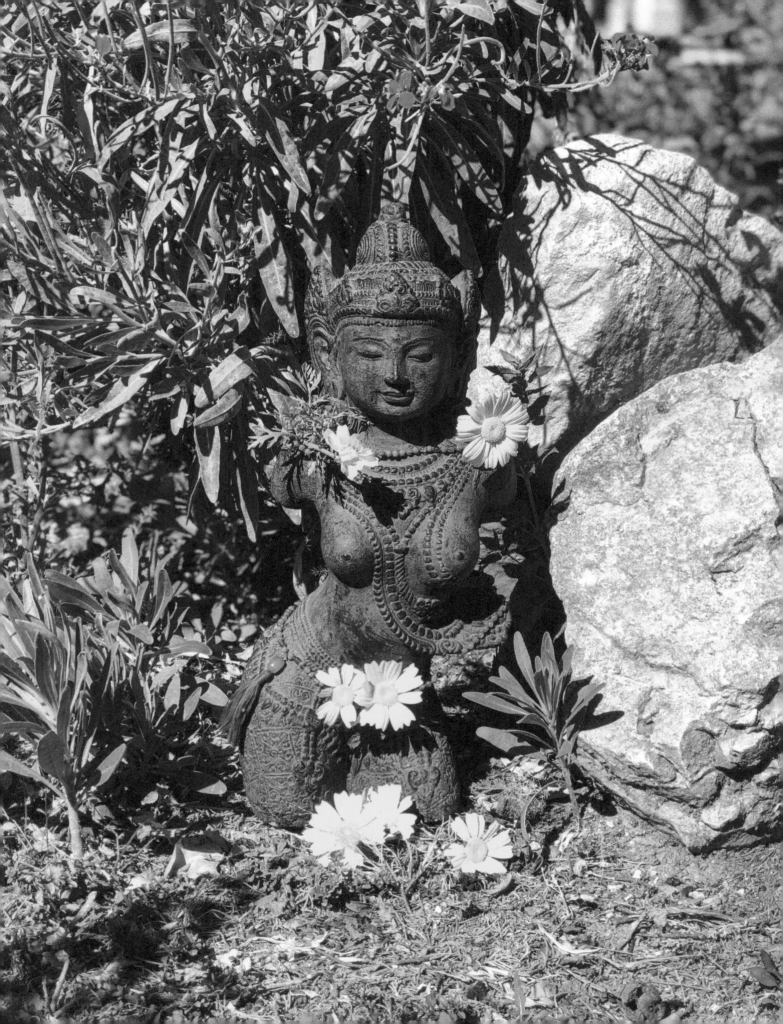

Conclusion

I hope that this guide gives an idea of **how amazing it has felt for me to learn more about the functioning of women's bodies**. Every day I thank my body for doing its best to stay in balance in an environment which is not always kind towards it. To better understand my anatomy and physiology has helped me look after myself better. **Our women's circle has shared with you many of the practical tips we use ourselves, and which we believe to be quite easy to integrate into your life, step by step, starting with the ones which resonate most with your current situation.**

We have also introduced you to holistic health systems which bring symptoms back into their context and consider them to be messages that deserve listening to, rather than trouble-shooters to be silenced. Yoga, traditional Chinese medicine, homeopathy and Ayurveda are not trying to replace "classic" Western medicine, but they can help numerous women to prevent, soften, or even heal chronic problems without causing harmful side effects. **Your body is your home, some would say your "soul's temple"; trust in your ability to look after yourself on a daily basis.**

Gratitude

The daily practise of gratitude (starting or ending your day by reminding yourself of all that makes your life beautiful) **is a simple and effective way to feel happier.**
This book obviously owes a lot to the experts I introduced you to in our women's circle: they accepted to share what they know in a condensed form, which does not do their wisdom justice. Feel free to contact them individually to find out more!

Thank you to the talented artists who gave colours and form to this book:
Elena Jarmosh for the anatomical illustrations and the layout, **Cecilia Cristolovean** for the studio photography, **Heather Whitehouse** and **Adèle Chrétien** for the exterior photos. Adèle also set up the Youtube channel and helps me with the Instagram account.
I thank my teachers of the Birthlight school, Françoise Freedman and Kirsteen Ruffell, as well as all the other yoga instructors who shared their wisdom with me, especially Françoise Galan, Claude Vallot, Dominique Casaux, Uma Dinsmore-Tuli, Mirjam Wagner, and Zhozeh Zarrindast.
Thanks to my "peer review committee": Valérie Reinhart, Nadège Lanvin, Julie Pons, and Stéfanie Lolivret, and obviously my mum.
Thank you **Sarah Burgess** for your patient editing of the English version of this book.

Thank you Laure Bouys and the team at Yogaconnect, who filmed the French full-length classes and host them on their platform.
Thank you to my friends Mirjam and David, who let me stay in their beautiful house so I could write in peace.
Thank you to all the women with whom I spoke about these issues over the years, especially those who come to my classes and workshops, where we share our experiences.
Last but not least, thank you to "El Gato", who is the Yang to my Yin.

Commented bibliography

Here is the list of the books I have used for inspiration and research whilst writing this book (apart from my three Birthlight training manuals, which are not sold separately from the courses). I have added a little description for each title, so that this bibliography can help you dive deeper into issues you are particularly interested in.

Avant Stover, Sara, *The Way of the Happy Woman: Living the Best Year of your life*. Based on her own story, explains how she healed her health issues by changing her lifestyle. Offers recipes, psychological techniques and yoga sequences (Yin and Vinayasa) organised around the four seasons.

Bihar School of Yoga, *Asana Pranayama Mudra Bandha*. One of the classic hatha yoga manuals and the one used in the Bihar School's teacher training courses. Describes practises and their benefits. A must-have resource for traditional yoga practitioners.

Bredesen, Dr Dale E., *The End of Alzheimer's*. A useful read for those of you who know that cognitive decline runs in their family, as Dr Bredesen pioneers a different approach to treating these conditions. Amongst other things, he explains the link between female hormones, digestion and brain health. His programme works, he has proven it. When people tell you there is nothing that can be done to treat these conditions, they are wrong.

de Gasquet, Dr Bernadette, *Périnée arrêtons le massacre*. This French gynaecologist and yoga teacher advocates birthing positions and strengthening exercises that don't damage the pelvic floor. This book explains the anatomical background of the pelvic floor really well and offers targeted exercises, in particular for the abdominal muscles.

Devi, Nischala Joy, *The Healing Path of Yoga*. After setting up the yoga part of Dr Dean Ornish's famous programme for a healthy heart, Nischala, a former monastic yogini, wrote this lovely book about healing through yoga, based on her experience with visualisations and adaptations of classic postures for fragile practitioners.

Dinsmore Tuli, Uma, *Yoni Shakti*. A wonderful tome of a book by an international yoga teacher who specialises in her teaching of "*womb yoga*", focusing on fertility, pregnancy and menopause. Whilst the historical and mythical part goes into great detail, this book also offers a wealth of interesting case studies from Uma's students. It presents several beautiful yoga nidras for the different milestones of a woman's life and quite original yoga sequences.

Enders, Giulia, *Gut, the inside story of our body's most under-rated organ*. This German medical student's international bestseller inspired an exhibition on the microbiome and encouraged millions of people to take a closer look at probiotics, microbes, and... poo. Her light tone and funny drawings help to explain a very serious subject.

Gray, Miranda, *Red Moon - Understanding and using the creative, sexual and spiritual gifts of the menstrual cycle*. The creator of the Womb Blessing ceremony explains the phases of the menstrual cycle, their influence on the feminine psyche, and how to organise your life to reap benefits from this awareness.

Hariri, Yuval Noah, *Sapiens*. The famous Israeli historian's best-known book retraces the entire history of human evolution. The part about the transition from a nomadic lifestyle to agriculture, then industrialisation, is particularly interesting for the topic of women's health.

Liedloff, Jean, *The Continuum Concept*. This book from the 1970s has left a deep impression on me. Mainly known for advocating baby holding and co-sleeping, there is much more to discover in this American woman's account of living in the jungle amongst people wrongly considered as "primitive".

Lukac, Rika, *Eat, Breathe, Conceive*. This practical guide by a Dutch yoga teacher and nutritionist does a marvellous job of explaining all the physiological aspects of fertility and offers a specific yoga sequence. The part about nutrition is very detailed and can seem overwhelming, but it is very thorough, and well-presented.

Noroc, Mihaela, *The Atlas of Beauty*. This is a gorgeous collection of photos depicting women whom Romanian photographer Mihaela met by chance whilst traveling the world. An extraordinary photography project which celebrates womanhood, diversity, and solidarity.

Northrup, Dr Christiane, *Women's Bodies, Women's wisdom, The complete guide to women's health and wellbeing*. This could be called the "bible" of women's health, a big fat book full of information and personal accounts form this American doctor who combines classic medicine with alternative healing methods. A must-have for every woman!

Rodrigues, Dinah, *Hormone Yoga Therapy for Women*. Brazilian yoga legend Dinah created a specific yoga therapy method which has proven effects on raising oestrogen and progesterone levels. Whilst there are some contraindications to her sequence (hormone-dependent cancers, endometriosis and hyperthyroidism, in particular) and it is a bit peculiar at times, it has helped many women conceive or navigate menopause.

Staugaard Jones, Jo Ann, *The Vital Psoas Muscle: Connecting Physical, Emotional, and Spiritual Wellbeing*. Yes, here is an entire book on the psoas – what it looks like, how it works, what it does, which chakras it is connected to, which yoga and Pilates exercises help it. Very specific, a really useful book, for back-pain and women's issues in particular.

Tiwari, Maya, *The Path of Practice: A Woman's Book of Healing with Food, Breath, and Sound*. This was a very important stepping stone on my own path as a woman and as a yoga teacher. Maya, who lived in New York City but had Indian ancestry, self-healed from cancer by using natural methods based on Ayurveda. She went on to found the Wise Earth school of Ayurveda. She teaches about the importance of food, of ritual, and of natural rhythms for women's health.

Uvnäs Moberg, Dr Kerstin, *The Hormone of Closeness - The Role of Oxytocin in Relationships*.

A fascinating book which explains the role of oxytocin in relations between mother and child, between lovers, and within groups. Detailed medical and sociological explanations, but easy to understand.

van Lysebeth, André, *Tantra, The Cult of the Feminine*. A really unique book (and difficult to find these days) by one of the first French-speaking yoga masters. It explains everything about Tantra. Whilst the first part is only of interest to yoga historians, the second part is very practical and offers exercises for men and women, in particular for the pelvic floor. His style may be a bit dated, yet this book remains an absolute reference.

Vitti, Alisa, *Womancode: Perfect Your Cycle, Amplify Your Fertility, Supercharge Your Sex Drive and Become a Power Source*. This is a useful reference to go deeper into some of the subjects mentioned in this book, such as acidity, blood sugar, the liver, the menstrual cycle. Alisa also described her own battle to heal her PCOS. Its opinions and methods can be quite extreme, but it is interesting.

Wagner, Mirjam, *YIN FOR LIFE - Nourishing guidance for women in all stages*, (upcoming). Mirjam blends into this wonderful book her personal experience and all the specific tools she has been using for over a decade to help women flourish: yin yoga, feminine archetypes, and an intimate knowledge of the human body, all inform this long-awaited compendium.

White, Jani, *The Fertile Fizz, Improve Your Chances of Conception by Reducing Stress, Improving Nutrition and Amplifying your Sexuality*. This is our acupuncture expert Jani's lovely book. The "very sexy biology lesson" offers an original and artistic approach based on years of clinical experience. It speaks to the couple and not just to the woman.

Wylde, Suzanne, *Moving Stretch*. Excellent guide to the fascia, which starts by explaining the theory, then offers simple specific stretches, especially to improve one's posture.

Online resources:

My website with the "animated photos" from this book to show you the poses "live": www.susanne-haegele.com and its accompanying **Youtube channel** of the same name.

Actionaid (www.actionaid.org.uk), a charity dedicated to fighting "period poverty" worldwide. From supporting Girls' Clubs that help girls learn about periods, to distributing sanitary kits in emergencies and training women to make cheap, reusable sanitary pads, they help to make sure every woman and girl can manage her period with dignity.

Birthlight (www.birthlight.com), **a training organisation which enables existing yoga teachers to further develop their skills and knowledge with a focus on pre- and postnatal yoga and women's wellbeing** ("*Wellwoman*"), founded by anthropologist and yoga teacher Françoise Freedman. Excellent trainings offered in Europe, Russia and China, and now globally online.

Endometriosis UK (www.endometriosis-uk.org), the UK-based charity dedicated to helping women affected by endometriosis by offering support services, reliable information and a community. They raise awareness, provide a helpline, and are involved in research.

Hilde Atalanta, The Vulva Gallery (www.hildeatalanta.com/thevulvagallery), and the.vulva.gallery on Instagram, artsy illustrations presenting the vulva in all its aspects. Sexual education and awareness are the goal, the presentation is cheeky and inclusive. The Vulva Gallery is a body positive platform and for all sexual orientations.

Mirjam Wagner's online studio (www.yogatherapymallorca.com/onlinestudio/), in English, offers beautifully produced videos taught by Mirjam herself, with Yin Yoga, feminine archetypes and hormones. She is currently working on an online course focusing on women's hormones. Also offers some of her daughter's beautiful poems.

Odile Fillod's website, creator of the 3D printable clitoris model as shown in this book's illustration (https://odilefillod.wixsite.com/clitoris).

Thrive Homeopathy, Sarah Davison's website, has a dedicated space for menopause issues and offers a targeted online programme for menopausal women (https://thrivehomeopathy.com/homeopathy-for-menopause/).

Yogaconnect (www.myyogaconnect.com), this wonderful French online yoga platform has many of my classes as video recordings, including the four sequences presented in this book (in French). The first two weeks of subscription are free.

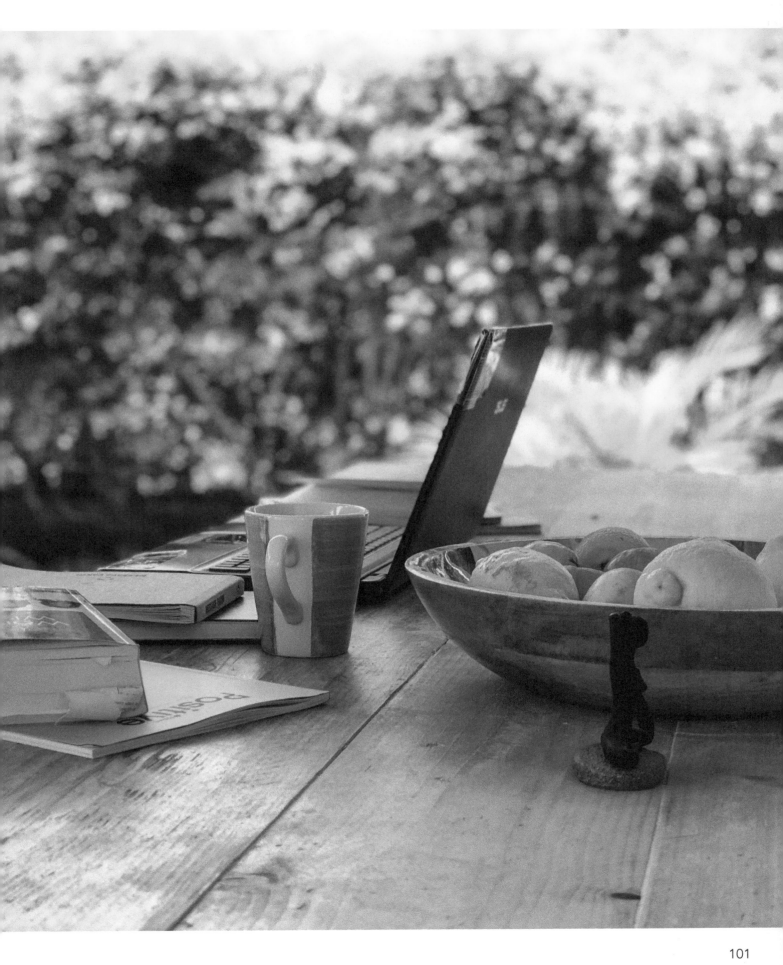

Index

Scientific sources

i Dr. Alyson McGregor specialises in this area and has written about it in *Sex Matters – how male-centric medicine endangers women's health and what to do about it*. See her website: https://www.alysonmcgregormd.com/book

ii UK Mental Health Foundation's "Sleep Matters" report, 2011, www.HowDidYouSleep.org

iii www.ncbi.nlm.nih.gov/pmc/articles/PMC3832324/

iv https://www.who.int/ipcs/publications/en/ch1.pdf?ua=1

v www.who.int/mediacentre/news/releases/2013/hormone_disrupting_20130219/fr/

vi https://hal-pasteur.archives-ouvertes.fr/pasteur-01349062/document

vii www.ncbi.nlm.nih.gov/pmc/articles/PMC5961632/

viii www.ncbi.nlm.nih.gov/pmc/articles/PMC2761884/

ix www.ncbi.nlm.nih.gov/pmc/articles/PMC5641835/

x www.ncbi.nlm.nih.gov/pubmed/26601965 , www.alternativesante.fr/alzheimer/alzheimer-parkinson-le-microbiote-intestinal-et-les-facteurs-environnementaux-en-premiere-ligne

xi www.ncbi.nlm.nih.gov/pmc/articles/PMC4566456/

xii www.ncbi.nlm.nih.gov/pmc/articles/PMC4841791/

xiii https://www.ncbi.nlm.nih.gov/pubmed/23662151 and https://www.ncbi.nlm.nih.gov/pubmed/16884344 and https://www.ncbi.nlm.nih.gov/pubmed/22435409 and many more.

xiv www.nih.gov/news-events/nih-research-matters/egg-producing-stem-cells-found-women

xv www.rbmojournal.com/article/S1472-6483(13)00007-2/fulltext

xvi www.ncbi.nlm.nih.gov/pubmed/29108503

xvii www.e-sante.fr/tampons-et-serviettes-des-residus-de-substances-chimiques-encore-presents/breve/615377

xviii See the description of Dr. Kegel's research in André van Lysebeth's Tantra book, and more recently: www.jsm.jsexmed.org/article/S1743-6095(17)31043-3/fulltext or https://www.psychologytoday.com/intl/blog/how-the-mind-heals-the-body/201412/the-stress-sex-connection

xix See Kerstin Uvnas-Moberg's book in the bibliography.

Lightning Source UK Ltd.
Milton Keynes UK
UKHW020734101120
373091UK00002B/3